Textbook of Fungal Infections

Textbook of Fungal Infections

Cristian Parker

AMERICAN
MEDICAL PUBLISHERS
www.americanmedicalpublishers.com

AMERICAN
MEDICAL PUBLISHERS
www.americanmedicalpublishers.com

Cataloging-in-publication Data

Textbook of fungal infections / edited by Cristian Parker.
p. cm.
Includes bibliographical references and index.
ISBN 979-8-88740-659-6
1. Mycoses. 2. Mycoses--Diagnosis. 3. Mycoses--Treatment.
4. Communicable diseases. 5. Infection. I. Parker, Cristian.
RC117 .F863 2023
616.969--dc23

American Medical Publishers,
41 Flatbush Avenue,
1st Floor, New York,
NY 11217, USA

ISBN 979-8-88740-659-6 (Hardback)

Contents

Preface

Fungal infections are diseases that are caused by fungus. They can affect the skin, nails, and lungs. Various types of fungal infections have been divided into three categories, namely superficial, subcutaneous, and systemic fungal infections. Subcutaneous fungal infections usually affect tissues beneath the skin, whereas systemic fungal infections can affect organs such as the lungs, eyes, liver, and brain. Some of the major fungal infections include athlete's foot, jock itch, pityriasis versicolor, ringworm, and thrush. The common symptoms of fungal infections vary widely and can include blisters, irritation, itching, redness, scaly skin, swelling, and difficulty in breathing. Immunocompromised people are at an increased risk of fungal infections. The diagnosis of fungal infections can be done using a combination of physical examination and laboratory tests, such as skin or blood cultures. After the type of fungal infection has been diagnosed, the medical practitioners usually prescribe a treatment involving antifungal medications, which may be administered orally or topically. The most common anti-fungal medications include azoles, polyenes, echinocandins, and allylamines. The patients should complete the full course of medicine prescribed to them to prevent the development of drug-resistant strains of the fungus. The topics covered in this extensive book deal with the core subject of fungal infections. It will provide comprehensive knowledge to the readers.

This book unites the global concepts and researches in an organized manner for a comprehensive understanding of the subject. It is a ripe text for all researchers, students, scientists or anyone else who is interested in acquiring a better knowledge of this dynamic field.

I extend my sincere thanks to the contributors for such eloquent research chapters. Finally, I thank my family for being a source of support and help.

Cristian Parker

Chapter 1

An Introduction to Fungi

Fungi

Fungus

A fungus is a eukaryote that digests food externally and absorbs nutrients directly through its cell walls. Most fungi reproduce by spores and have a body (thallus) composed of microscopic tubular cells called hyphae. Fungi are heterotrophs and, like animals, obtain their carbon and energy from other organisms. Some fungi obtain their nutrients from a living host (plant or animal) and are called biotrophs; others obtain their nutrients from dead plants or animals and are called saprotrophs (saprophytes, saprobes). Some fungi infect a living host, but kill host cells in order to obtain their nutrients; these are called necrotrophs.

Age of Fungi

Fungi are an ancient group—not as old as bacteria, which fossil evidence suggests may be 3. 5 billion years old—but the earliest fungal fossils are from the Ordovician, 460 to 455 million years old.

Economic Importance of Fungi

The fungi are of great economic importance on account of their both harmful as well as beneficial effects. A large number of fungi cause destructive havoc to our valuable crop and timber plants, various lines of food products. They also attack the live-stock as well as human beings. But, all of them are not harmful to the mankind, as most of the species bring about decomposition of dead bodies of plants and animals as well as of animal dung.

The harmful economic aspects of fungi are as follows:

- Spoilage of food, stored grains and other essential commodities: Fungi (mould fungi) are the chief agents responsible for most of the disintegration of fruits, vegetables and other done stuffs, e.g. jams, jelly, pickles, bread, various cooked-foods eat. If not properly stored. Common food damaging fungi are Aspergillus, Penicillium, Mucor and Rhizopus. About 25 -50% of harvested fruits and vegetables are destroyed by fungi.
- Induce diseases of plants: Fungi are also responsible for millions of rupees worth of damage to crops by causing plast diseases. Of the serious diseases of crop plants, late blight disease of potato plant caused by Phytophthora infestans; Claviceps purpurea (Ascomycotina) causes the 'ergot' disease of rye. The members of 'rust' (Puccinia) and 'smut' (Ustilago, Tilletia, etc.) are also highly destructive to various different crop plants like wheat, maize, oct, barley etc. Many fungi cause immense loss to timber trees by causing wood-rot disease.

- Induce diseases of animals and human being: Fungi are responsible for the diseases of animals as well as human beings. Some of the serious diseases of human being, i.e. the diseases of skin, far, throat, nose and as well as bronchial and intestinal disorders are caused by various groups of fungi. A few species of Mucor and Rhizopus are common fungi infecting lungs, brain and gastric system, Neurospora and Fusarium infect corneal tissue of eye. Several species of Aspergillus are human pathogens, causing a group of diseases collectively called Aspergilloses.
- Toxic substances obtained from fungi: Several toxins have been extracted from mushroom like Amantia phalloides, Aspergillus flavous and Aspergillus niger may infest dried foods and ground out meal and produce a dangerous toxins called aflatoxin - this toxin has carginogenic effect.
- Wood-rotting fungi: Many wood rotting fungi e.g. a few species of Lentinus, Serpula lacrymans, Coniophora cerebella, etc. cause a great monetary loss. Dry rot and wet rot are most dangerous diseases of the timber.
- Fungi growing in Aircraft fuel tanks: *Amorphotheca resinae* is the main organism of the kerosene-based fuel tanks of aircrafts. This fungus grows in storage and fuel tanks profusely as result fungal hyphae may plug the valves and pipes of the aircraft and cause disastrous effect during flight.

Meaning of Fungi

Fungi are eukaryotic organisms that include microorganisms such as yeasts, moulds and mushrooms. These organisms are classified under kingdom fungi.

The organisms found in Kingdom fungi contain a cell wall and are omnipresent. They are classified as heterotrophs among the living organisms.

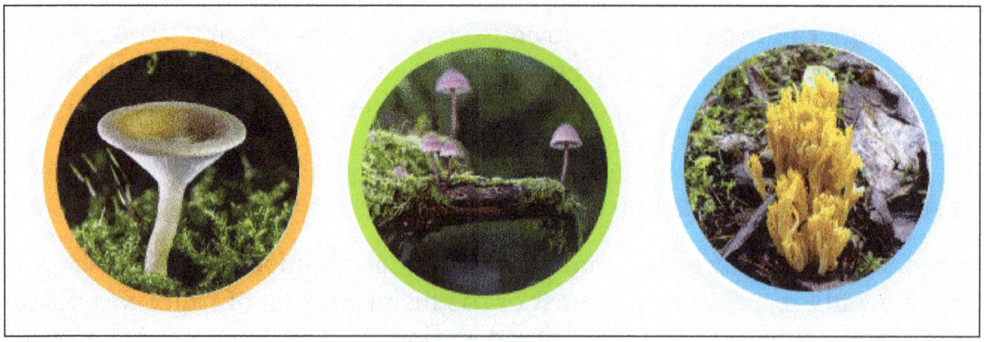

Kingdom Fungi

To name a few – the appearance of black spots on bread left outside for some days, the mushrooms and the yeast cells, which are commonly used for the production of beer and bread are also fungi. They are also found in most skin infections and other fungal diseases.

If we observe carefully, all the examples that we cited involve moist conditions. Thus, we can say that fungi usually grow in places which are moist and warm enough to support them.

Let us have a detailed overview of the structure, classification and characteristics of fungi.

Structure of Fungi

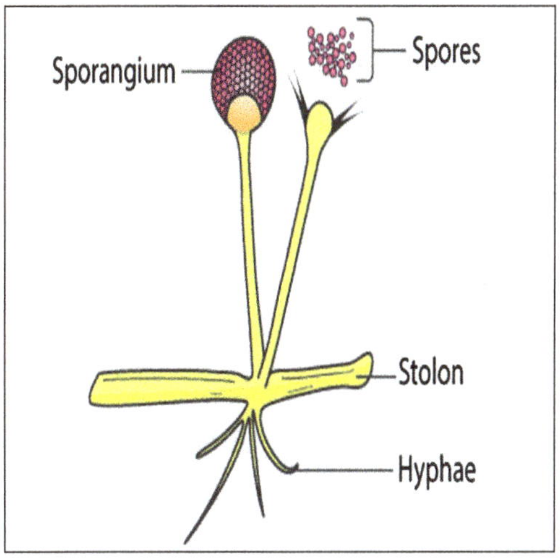

The structure of fungi can be explained in the following points:

- Almost all the fungi have a filamentous structure except the yeast cells.
- They can be either single-celled or multicellular organisms.
- Fungi consist of long thread-like structures known as hyphae. These hyphae together form a mesh-like structure called mycelium.
- Fungi possess a cell wall which is made up of chitin and polysaccharides.
- The cell wall comprises a protoplast, which is differentiated into other cell parts such as cell membrane, cytoplasm, cell organelles and nuclei.
- The nucleus is dense, clear, with chromatin threads. The nucleus is surrounded by a nuclear membrane.

Characteristics of Fungus

General features of fungi:

- Fungi are cosmopolitan in nature.
- They are eukaryotic.
- They are heterotrophic in nutrition.
- They may be saprophytes, parasite or symbionts.
- Thallus may be plasmodium, pseudoplsmodium or mycelia.
- They may be unicellur or filamentous multicellular.

- Cell wall is primarily composed of chitin and glucans, although the walls of some species contain cellulose.
- They lack chlorophyll pigments and are incapable of photosynthesis.
- Life cycle may be simple to complex.
- Reproduce by sexually, asexually, parasexually.

Morphological characteristics of fungi:

Characters	Remarks
Eukaryotic	Possess membrane-bound nuclei (containing chromosomes) and a range of membrane-bound cytoplasmic organelles (e.g. mitochondria, vacuoles, endoplasmic reticulum).
Distribution	Cosmopolitan
Habit	May be free-living or may form intimate relationships with other organisms i.e. free-living, parasitic or mutualistic (symbiotic).
Filamentous/Unicellular	Most are filamentous, composed of individual microscopic filaments called hyphae, which exhibit apical growth and which branch to form a network of hyphae called a mycelium. Some are unicellular: e.g. yeasts.
Thallus	Plasmodial, pseudoplasmodial, pseudomycelial,mycelial.
Cell Wall	Composed primarily of chitin and glucans, although the walls of some species contain cellulose (Oomycetes).
Nuclear Status	Multinucleate, homo or heterokaryotic, haploid (n), diploid (2n), dikaryotic (n + n).
Achlorophyllous	They lack chlorophyll pigments and are incapable of photosynthesis
Chemoheterotrophic (chemoorganotrophic)	They utilise pre-existing organic sources of carbon in their environment and the energy from chemical reactions to sythesise the organic compounds they require for growth and energy.
Storage compounds	Trehalose, glycogen, sugar alcohols and lipids.
Life cycle	Simple and complex
Reproduction	Sexual, asexual, parasexual reproduction often result in the production of spores.

General Characteristics of Fungi

Some of the most important characters of fungi are as follows:

- Occurrence,
- Thallus organization,
- Different forms of mycelium,
- Cell structure,
- Nutrition,

- Heterothallism and Homothallism,
- Reproduction.

Occurrence:

- Fungi are cosmopolitan and occur in air, water soil and on plants and animals.
- They prefer to grow in warm and humid places. Hence, we keep food in the refrigerator to prevent bacterial and fungal infestation.

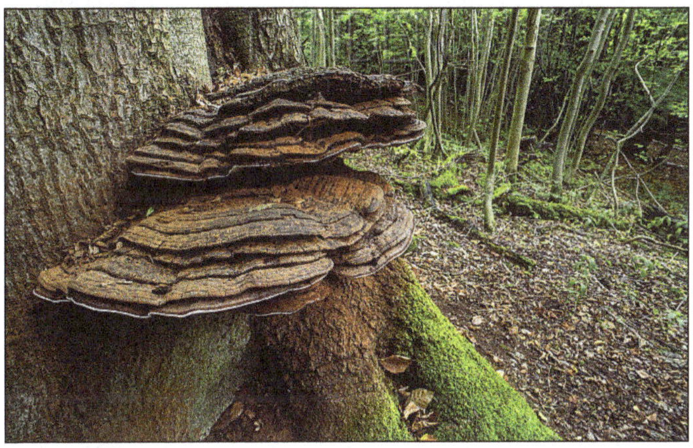

Thallus organization:

- Except some unicellular forms (e.g. yeasts, Synchytrium), the fungal body is a thallus called mycelium.
- The mycelium is an interwoven mass of thread-like hyphae (Sing, hypha). Hyphae may be septate (with cross wall) and aseptate (without cross wall). Some fungi are dimorphic that found as both unicellular and mycelial forms e.g. Candida albicans.
- The thallus may be two types: Unicellular and filamentous.

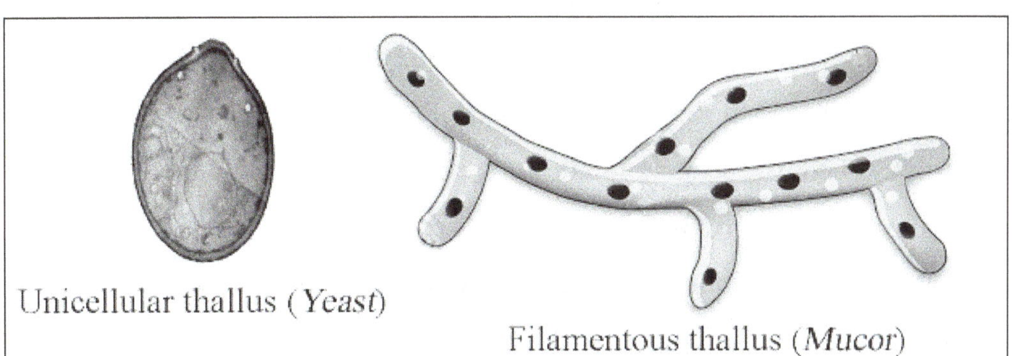

- Unicellular thallus: In some of the lower fungi, thallus is more or less a spherical, single celled structure. At the time of reproduction it becomes a reproductive unit. Such fungi are called holocarpic. In the unicellular holocarpic forms, the mycelium is absent e.g. Synchytrium. Some holocarpic fungi (e.g., yeast) producing bud cells in succession and these remain attached to one another in a chain. Such a chain of bud cells is referred to as pseudomycelium.

- Filamentous thallus: In most true fungi, the thallus is filamentous composed of Hyphae. Loosely aggregated hyphae are collectively forms a network known as mycelium. Each hypha may vary in shapes and sizes. Branching of hyphae is dichotomous. On the basis of presence or absence of septa the hyphae of mycelical fungi are of two types:
    - Nonseptate or aseptate hyphae: Mycelium contains numerous nuclei,lying in a common mass of cytoplasm, without cross wall in the hyphae, E.g., oomycetes and zygomycetes. Such a condition is known as coenocytic. However, septa may be laid down at the time of formation of reproductive organs to delimit them from the rest of the vegetative hyphae, therefore called Pseudosepta. E.g., Allomyces.
    - Septate Hyphae: Hyphae are septate and hyphal segments may contain one, two or more nuclei. E.g., Ascomycotina, Basidiomycotina, and Deuteromycotina. There are two types of septa:
- Primary septa: Primary septa are formed in association with mitotic or meiotic nuclear division, and they separate the daughter nuclei. These types of septa are found in Ascomycotina, Basidiomycotina and their asexual states.
- Adventitious septa: Adventitious septa are formed in the absence of mitosis or meiosis and occur especially in association with change in the local concentration of cytoplasm. These are found in lower groups of fungi as mastigomycotina and zygomycotina.

Following are the important characteristics of fungi:

- Fungi are eukaryotic, non-vascular, non-motile and heterotrophic organisms.
- They may be unicellular or filamentous.
- They reproduce by means of spores.
- Fungi exhibit the phenomenon of alternation of generation.
- Fungi lack chlorophyll and hence cannot perform photosynthesis.
- Fungi store their food in the form of starch.
- Biosynthesis of chitin occurs in fungi.
- The nuclei of the fungi are very small.
- The fungi have no embryonic stage. They develop from the spores.
- The mode of reproduction is sexual or asexual.
- Some fungi are parasitic and can infect the host.
- Fungi produce a chemical called pheromone which leads to sexual reproduction in fungi.
- Examples include mushrooms, moulds and yeast.

Important Terms in Mycology

Clinical mycology remains more of a descriptive art than an analytical science. You may find that the identification of fungi requires a greater development of your visual acuity than was necessary in bacteriology. There are also fewer biochemical tests available to aid in the differential identification of fungi. As a result you will spend considerable time in the laboratory visually examining fungal cultures. You will identify characteristic fungal structures by observing colonial growth both macroscopically and microscopically.

A thorough understanding of correct fungal terminology is of critical importance. You may find that the terms used to describe fungi are unusual, at times redundant, and often very confusing. We have attempted to simplify the jumbled jargon by providing you with the following list of terms that will be used most often in the laboratory section of this course. Although most of these terms have already been introduced in the lecture notes, they have been included in the laboratory manual as well.

Arthrospores - asexual, thick-walled spores formed by hyphal septation. Arthrospores are released only by fragmentation of the hyphae. The barrel-shaped arthrospores of Coccidioides immitis are the infectious stage of coccidioidomycosis.

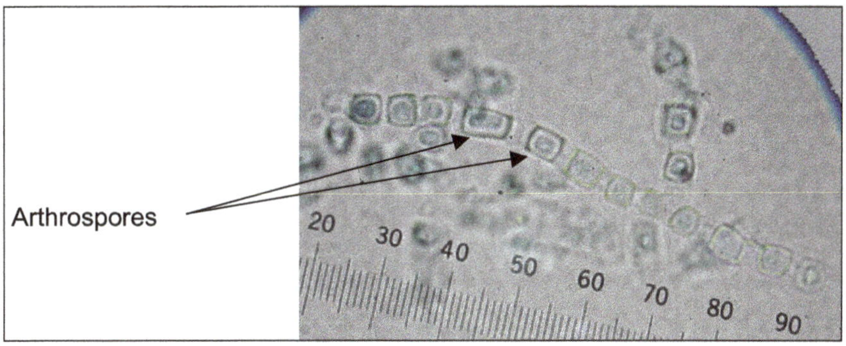

Chlamydospore - thick, double-walled, resistant, asexual spores that form as enlarged segments either within (intercalary) or at the tip (terminal) of hyphae. Often form under specific nutritional conditions where other spores do not form.

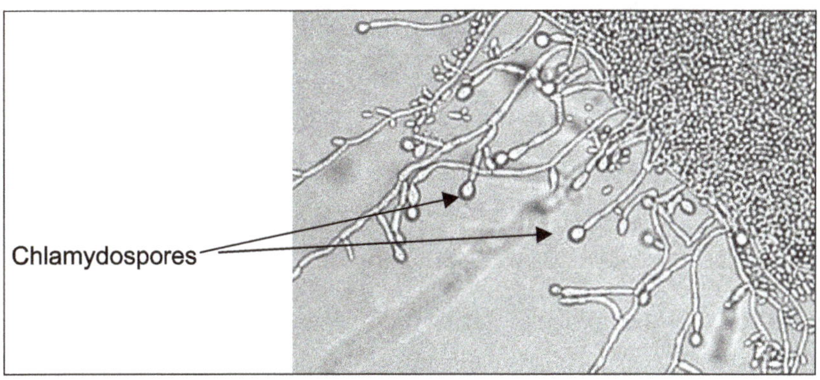

Conidia (singular = conidium) - asexual spores borne externally on hyphae or on a conidiophore; may be unicellular (microconidia) or multicellular (macroconidia).

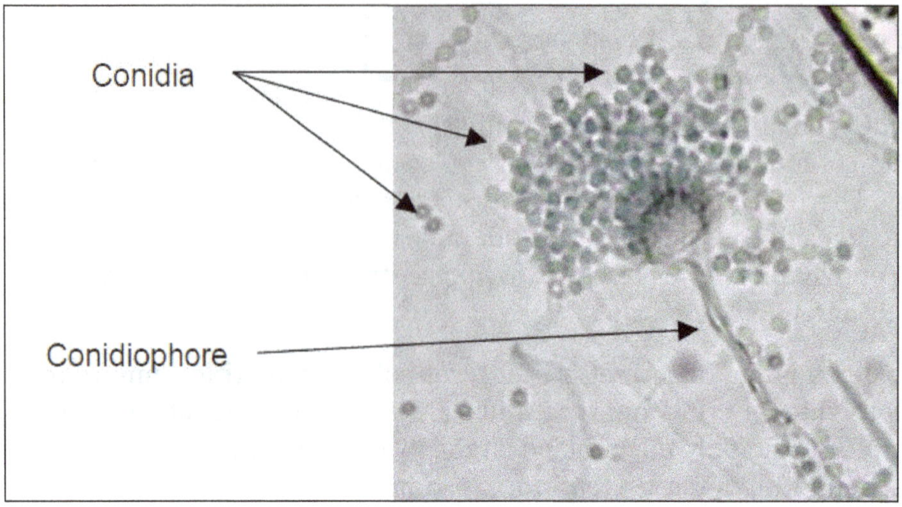

Conidiophore - the specialized hyphal stalk on which conidia develop either singly or in clusters.

Dematiaceous - dark-colored (green, brown, or black) fungi whose hyphae are pigmented. Both the top and the underside of the mycelia will be dark.

Dimorphic - Having both yeast and a mold (mycelial) form. Many of the systemic fungal pathogens are dimorphic.

Ectothrix - Dermatophytes that produce a sheath of arthrospores on the external surface of the hair shaft.

Endothrix - Dermatophytes that produce arthrospores within the hair shaft.

Endospore - Asexual spores formed within a cell (as in the spherule of Coccidioides immitis).

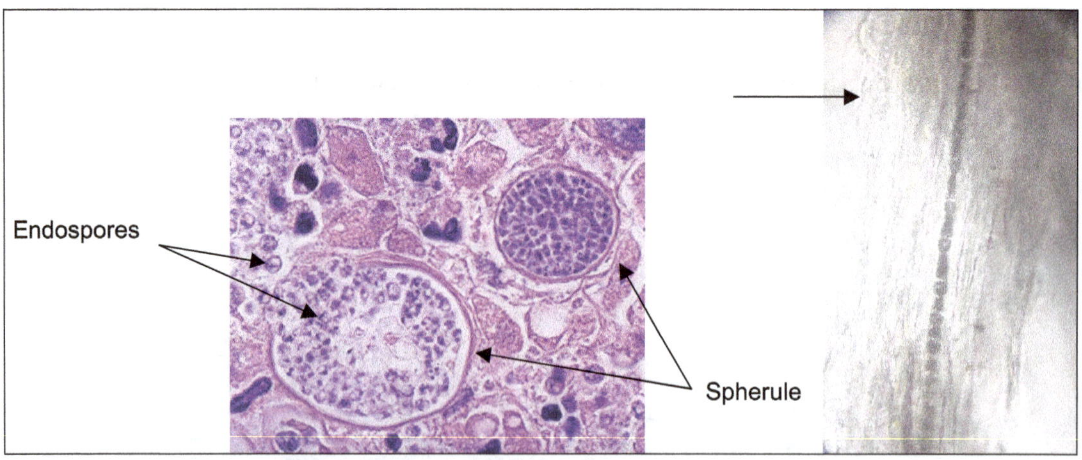

Geophilic - Refers to fungi whose natural habitat is the soil. Use of this term is generally restricted to certain Dermatophytes (e.g. Microsporum gypseum).

Germ-tube - The initial hyphal outgrowth of a germinating spore or yeast; especially important for identification of Candida albicans.

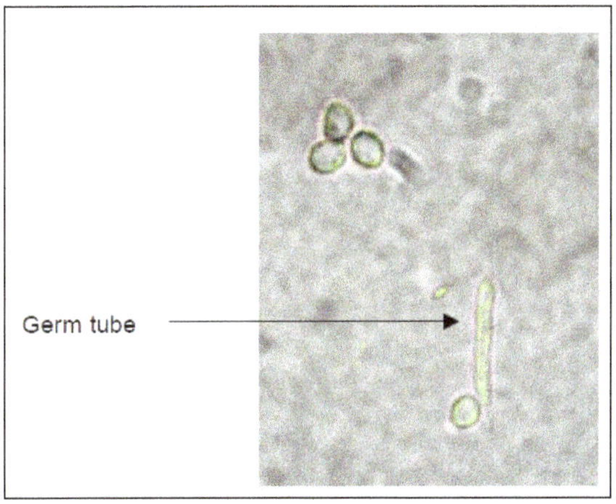

Mycelium - the intertwined mass of hyphae that forms the mold colony. The vegetative mycelium is composed of those hyphae that adhere to the substrate and absorbs nutrients. The aerial mycelium is composed of those hyphae that grow up from the surface and support the spores.

Pseudohyphae - chains of successively budding yeast cells that have complete cell walls, but have not detached from one another.

Rhizoid - rootlike branched hyphae which anchor the mycelium to the substrate; characteristic of certain Zygomycetes (Rhizopus and Absidium).

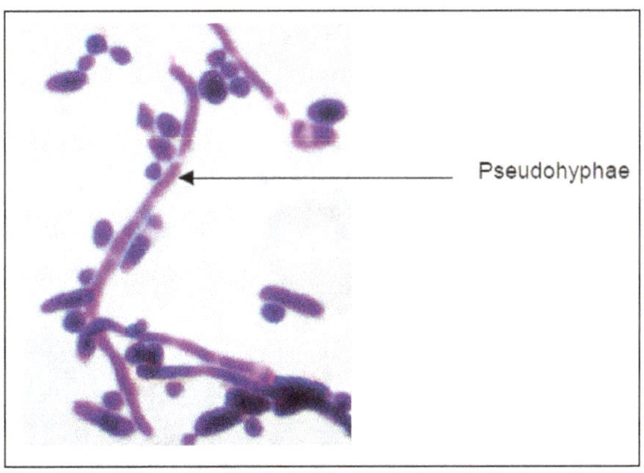

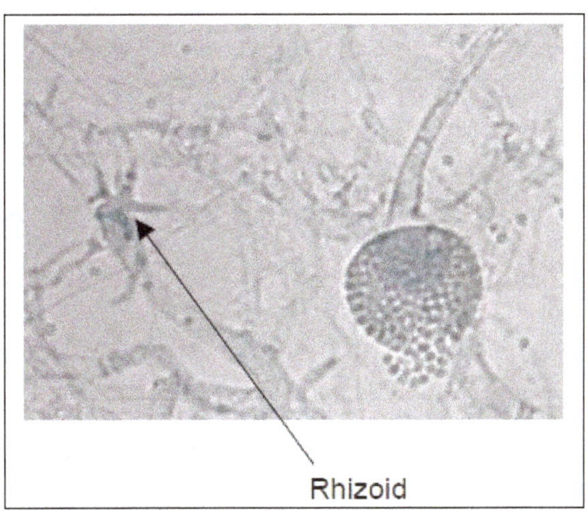

Septate - Cross-walls (septae) that divide hyphae into segments. If there are few or no cross-walls the hyphae are considered to be aseptate.

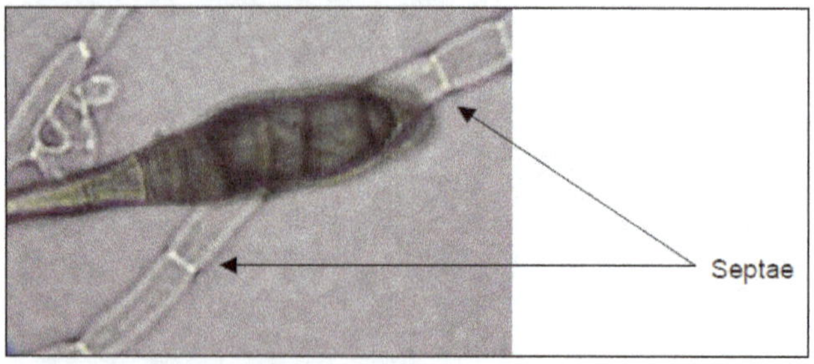

Sporangia (singular = sporangium)-spherical sack within which asexual spores (sporangiospores) form by progressive cytoplasmic cleavage.

Sporangiophore - specialized hyphal stalk which bears sporangia.

Sporangiospores - small spores contained within sporangia.

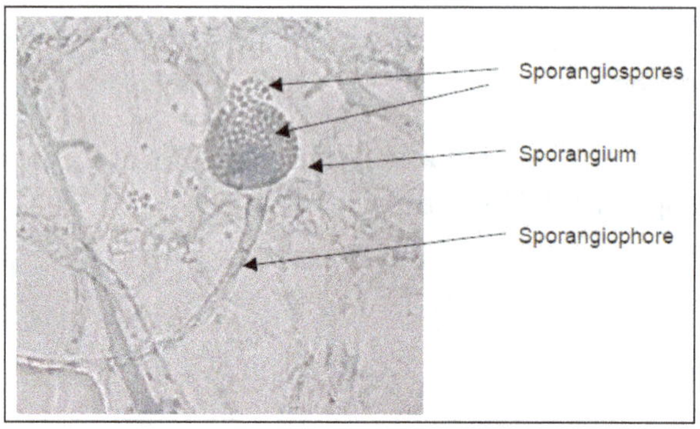

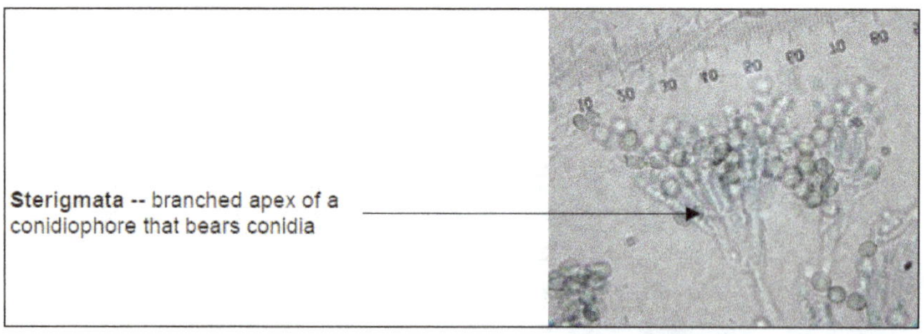

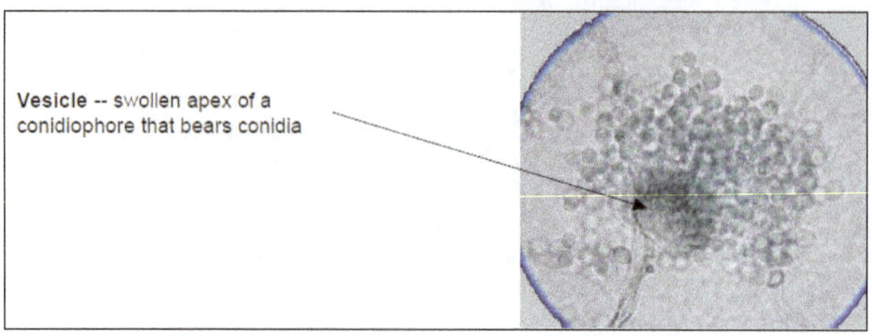

Zoophilic - refers to certain Dermatophytes that predominantly infect animals as opposed to humans (ex: Microsporum canis).

Identification of Fungal Organisms

Zygomycetes

Zygomycetes are rapidly growing molds that typically produce abundant hyphae that look like cotton candy and fill the air space in the tube or plate. They grow very rapidly (perhaps within 1-2 days) both at room temperature and at 37°C (thermotolerant). The Zygomycetes are distinguished from all other fungi by their production of broad, ribbonlike hyphae that usually have few or no septae (cross-walls) that can be seen microscopically. Some species have root-like hyphal extensions that anchor the hyphae. Also protruding from the hyphae are sporangiophores. The sporangiophores bear sac-like structures called sporangia that are filled with small sporangiospores.

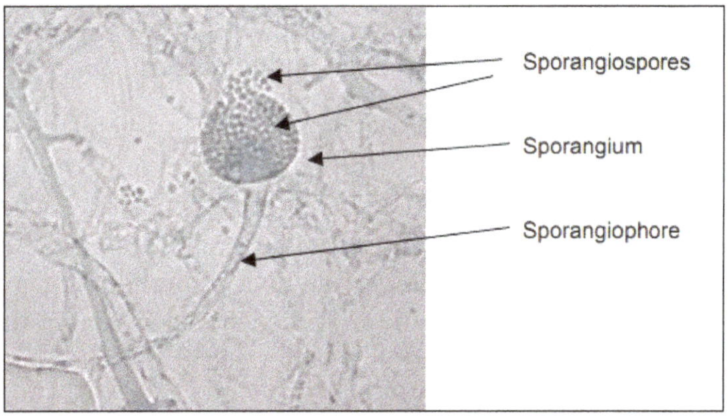

Absidia is the representative of the Zygomycetes we will look at in this laboratory microscopically. Other genera of this group that can be opportunistic pathogens include Rhizopus and Mucor. All of these molds look similar macroscopically. They can be distinguished microscopically by the presence (or absence) and position of rhizoids. The rhizoids of Absidia, are positioned between sporangiophores whereas they are found directly below the sporangiophores in Rhizopus. Mucor doesn't have rhizoids. You will not be expected to differentiate these organism based on rhizoid morphology.

Dematiaceous Molds

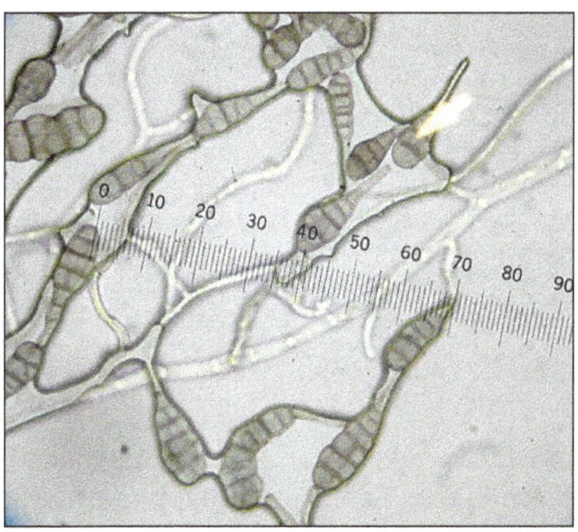

The term dematiaceous refers to molds whose hyphae are pigmented. Because of the pigment, the colonies of these fungi will appear dark green, brown, or black on both the top and reverse (underside). We will provide you with an isolate of Alternaria as an example of this group of fungi. Although it is hardly ever associated with infection, it is a very common contaminant, especially in specimens collected in the barn. Note the "hand-grenade" shape of the pigmented macroconidia. Other opportunistic pathogens of the dematiaceous group include Cladosporium, Phialophora, and Drechslera.

Hyaline Molds

Hyaline molds are fast-growing fungi that are common contaminants and occasional opportunistic pathogens. Some of these fungi can be relatively common and virulent pathogens (for example Aspergillus fumigatus in birds). Examples of opportunistic pathogens in this group include Pseudallescheria boydii, Aspergillus sp., Penicillium sp., and Fusarium sp.

Macroscopically, the colonies of these molds are lightly pigmented or non-pigmented. They may be white, light grey, green or light brown. The color is seen chiefly on top of the colony and is due to pigment in the many spores that are produced, not the hyphae. The hyphae are colorless (hyaline) and are septate. These organisms have hyphal projections called conidiophores. Some conidiophores terminate in either a swollen vesicle or a branched sterigmata. The vesicle and sterigmata bear abundant spores called conidia. These structures as a unit are sometimes referred to as "fruiting heads" or "fruiting bodies." Other conidiophores bear conidia singly or in small clusters.

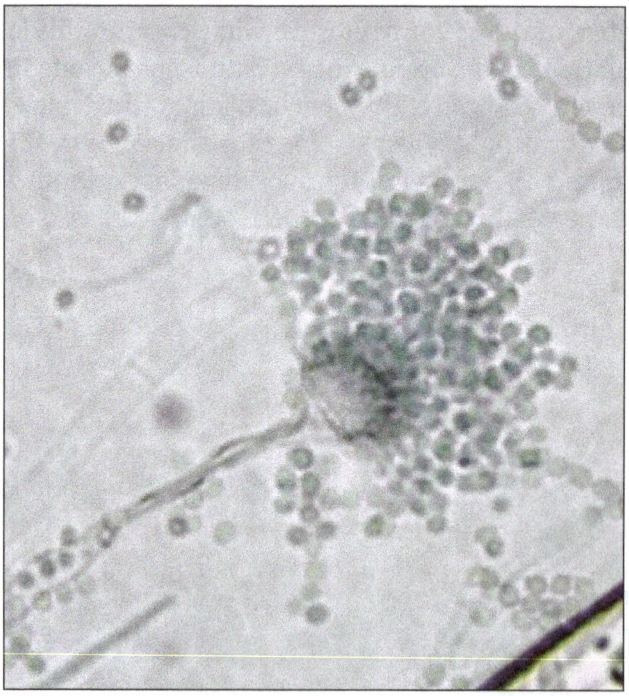

Aspergillus colonies are often white, grey, or green. They may also be yellow, tan, or brown. The colonies of Aspergillus niger are black. The septate hyphae of Aspergillus sp. produce conidiophores which terminate in swollen vesicles that bear chains of conidia.

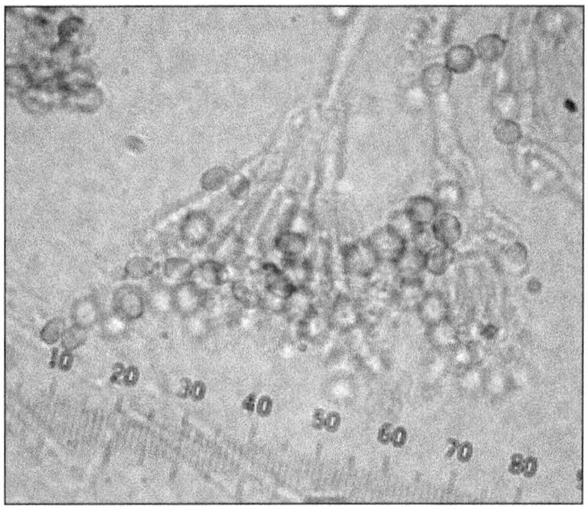

Most colonies of Penicillium sp. are some shade of green, but grey, yellow, orange, pink, or white colors may be encountered. The surface of the colonies is powdery because of the huge numbers of conidia. The septate hyphae of Penicillium sp. produce conidiophores which terminate in branched sterigmata that bear conidia.

The colonies of Fusarium sp. are cottony and have a distinctive lavender color. Their hyphae are septate and produce both macroconidia and microconidia. The microconidia are oval. The macroconidia are banana-shaped and multi-cellular. Typically, the macroconidia are produced in small clusters.

The colonies of Pseudallescheria boydii have a low, cottony surface that appears within 2-6 days. Unlike many hyaline molds, it will grow on mycobiotic agar. The septate hyphae produce single conidia that resemble lollipops. These lollipop conidia are similar to those produced by an important fungal pathogen, Blastomyces dermatitidis. Fortunately, Blastomyces can be converted to yeast at 37° while P. boydii cannot.

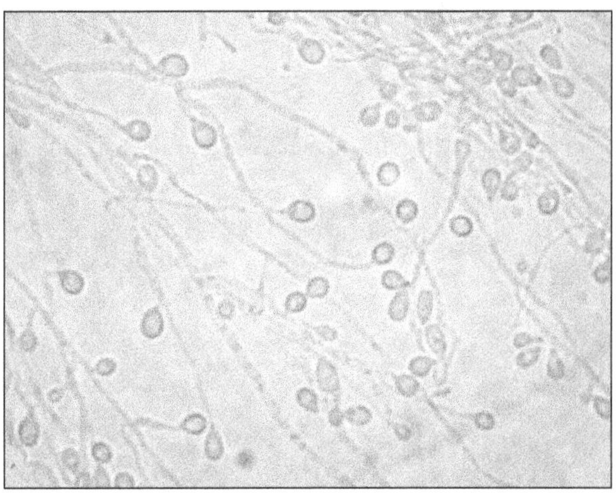

Yeasts

The colonial and microscopic appearance of yeasts differs greatly from that of molds. They grow somewhat more rapidly and may prefer to grow at warmer temperatures (35-37°C) than room temperature. Unlike molds, they do not have a fuzzy colonial appearance because they do not produce hyphae. Yeast colonies are flat and creamy in consistency, similar to many bacterial colonies. They grow a little more slowly, may become a little larger, and may have a more dense convex colonial appearance than bacterial colonies.

Microscopically, yeasts are larger than bacteria and can be visualized easily at 400x magnification (40x objective). Yeasts reproduce by budding - the cell wall projects outward to form a new daughter cell that eventually pinches off from the mother cell. Some may not separate entirely while budding, forming chains of unseparated yeast cells called pseudohyphae.

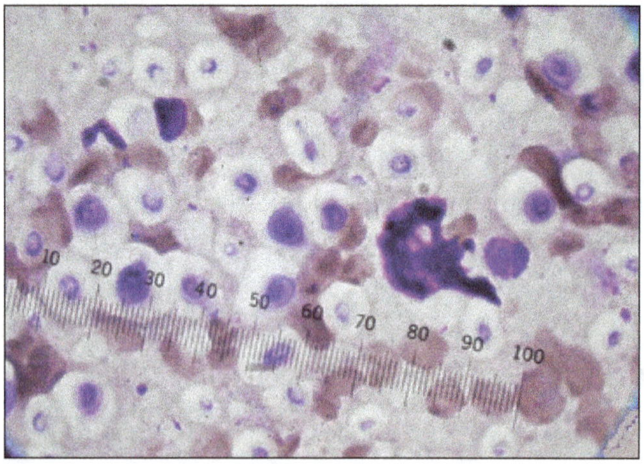

Cryptococcus neoformans produces mucoid colonies on Sabouraud agar and brain-heart infusion agar. Microscopically, these organisms are seen as budding yeasts with a narrow neck connecting the mother and daughter yeast cells. The production of a large, mucoid capsule is a unique feature of Cryptococcus among fungal organisms.

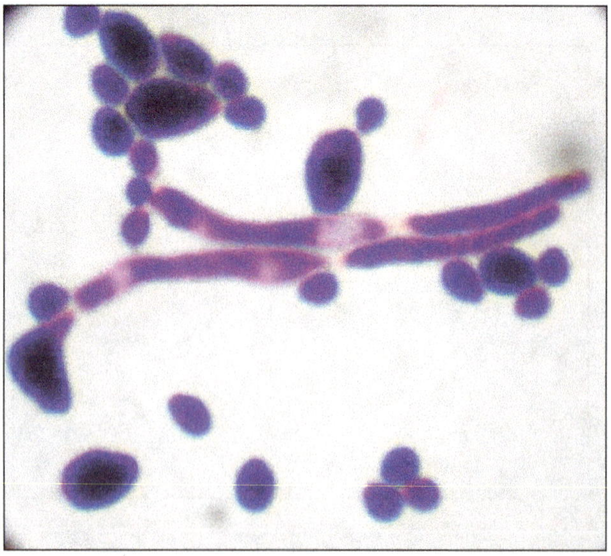

Candida albicans colonies have a buttery-like consistency on mycobiotic agar. Microscopically, Candida is composed principally of yeast cells, with occasional strings of unseparated budding yeast cells (pseudohyphae), and short structures resembling hyphae.

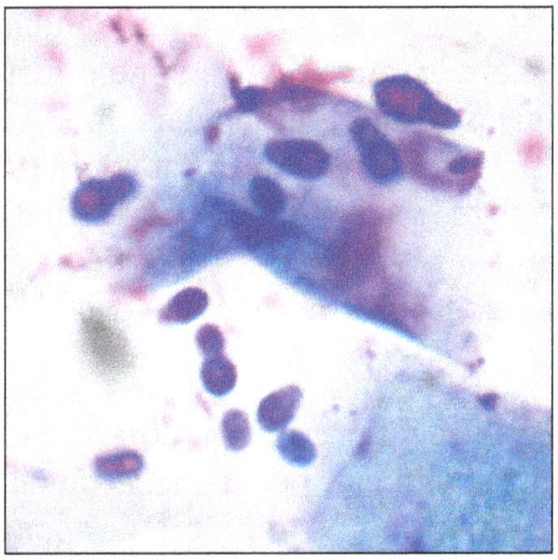

Malassezia pachydermatis (also called Pityrosporum) is a very common cause of otitis externa in dogs, especially those with heavy, floppy ears. We don't often culture it in our clinical laboratory because it is so easy to diagnose from clinical specimens. Ears infected with this organism have a characteristic bad smell. Microscopically, the organisms are oval or shaped like snowshoes or bowling pins. Somewhat surprisingly, there is rarely an inflammatory reaction in these cases, although a lot of brown discharge is produced that contains yeast organisms, squamous epithelial cells, and cerumen.

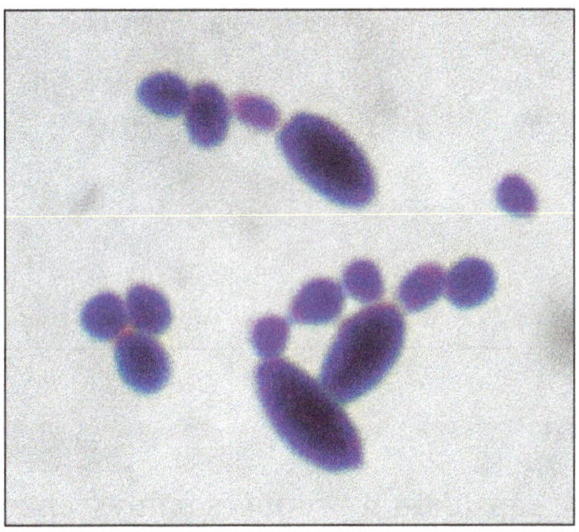

Other yeasts, like Saccharomyces - worshipped by many veterinary medical students for its role in the production of beer are nonpathogenic. They produce white to tan colonies that have a smooth, buttery appearance. Microscopically, they consist of single or budding yeasts. Prepare a Gram stain of Saccharomyces and compare its microscopic morphology to that of

Dimorphic Fungi

This class of fungi is characterized by two forms of growth:

1. Growth as a mold with septate hyphae in their natural reservoir (e.g. soil) or when incubated at 25° C. on conventional fungal media (Sabouraud dextrose or potato dextrose agars).
2. Growth as a yeast in the tissues of an animal/person or when incubated at 37° on enriched media (Brain heart infusion agar).

Compare the macroscopic colonial appearances of the yeast and mold forms of the organisms. The yeast forms have more of a moist appearance than the mold forms. The distinction is not always obvious, however, as the mold forms of these pathogens do not usually produce abundant aerial hyphae and therefore may lack the fuzzy appearance of common molds. In addition, conversion to the yeast form is often incomplete, resulting in cultures that have characteristics of both the mold and yeast forms of the organism. We will only provide the mold form of C. immitis because it is rather difficult to induce the yeast form of Coccidioides immitis in the laboratory because it requires increased levels of CO_2.

Although the colonial morphology of the dimorphs is rather nondescript, the microscopic appearance of these organisms, especially in clinical specimens, is much more useful in identifying them. The following pages include descriptions of the microscopic appearance of these dimorphic organisms.

Blastomyces Dermatitidis

The mold form of Blastomyces dermatitidis produces single "lollipop" conidia directly from the septate hyphae or delicate conidiophores. The yeast forms from clinical specimens are big, broad-based budding yeast cells with thick, double walls.

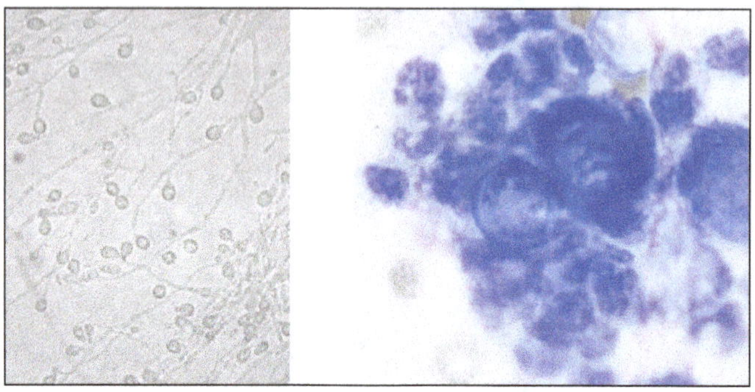

Histoplasma Capsulatum

The mold form of Histoplasma capsulatum produces spiny, tuberculate macroconidia that form on narrow conidiophores. They resemble the steering wheel of an old-fashioned ship like the Mayflower or an expensive yacht. Microconidia are rare. The yeast forms seen in clinical specimens are small, single-celled or budding yeasts present within macrophages.

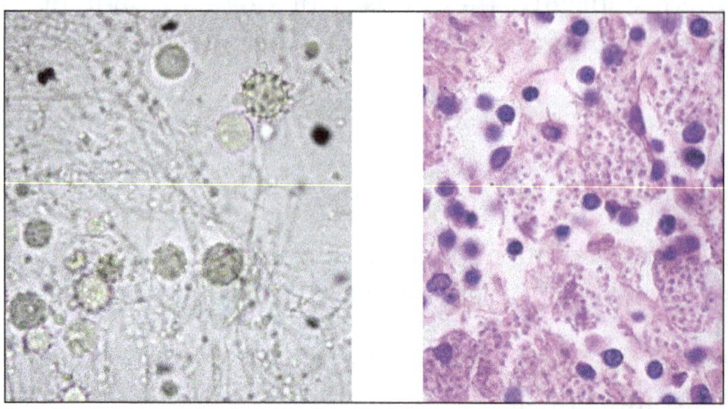

Coccidioides Immitis

The mold form of Coccidioides immitis produces barrel-shaped arthrospores which are formed by fragmentation of the hyphae. The arthrospores are the infectious form of the organism. The yeast forms seen in clinical specimens are huge spherules that contain numerous small endospores.

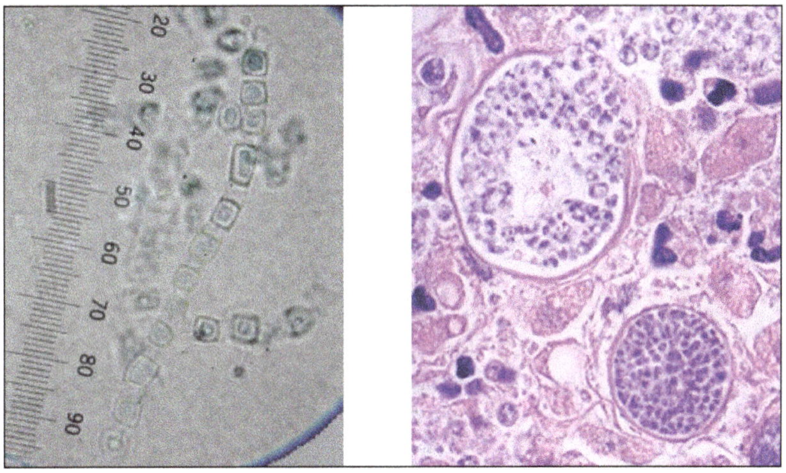

Sporothrix Schenckii

The mold form of Sporothrix schenckii produces thin, branching hyphae with delicate conidiopheres that bear clusters of small teardrop-shaped conidia at their tips. They resemble flowers on delicate stems. The yeast forms seen in clinical specimens are cigarshaped cells that are also known as "cigar bodies." The inflammatory reaction sometimes seen in the body is called an asteroid body.

Dimorphic Fungi

Microsporum Canis

The septate hyphae of Microsporum canis produce large, thick-walled, multi-septate, canoe-shaped macroconidia. Single macroconidia are borne directly from the hyphae or by attachment to a specialized cell. Microconidiospores are sparse if present at all.

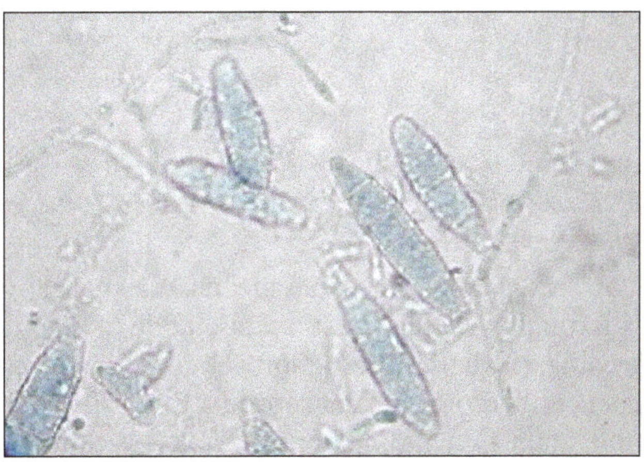

Microsporum Gypseum

The septate hyphae of Microsporum gypseum produce large macroconidia that are similar to those of Microsporum canis except that they are rowboat-shaped with more rounded ends. Microconidia are conspicuously absent.

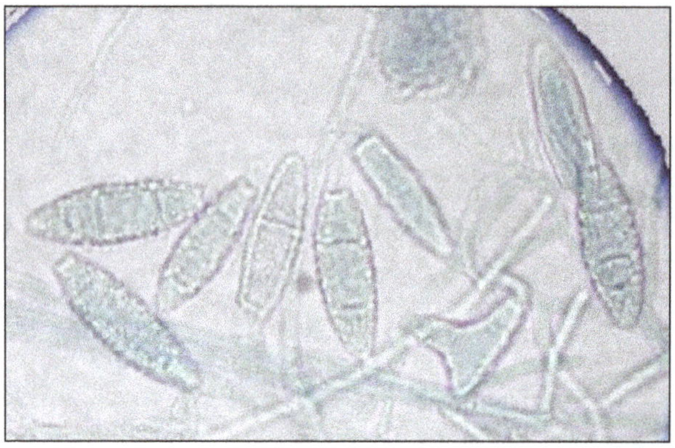

Trichophyton sp.

The septate hyphae of Trichophyton produce numerous small microconidia that form along the sides of the hyphae in clusters. Macroconidia are similar to those of Microsporum sp. except that they are cigar-shaped and have thinner, smoother walls. They are also quite rare, so don't spend a lot of time looking for them. If you are lucky enough to find one, let the rest of us know!

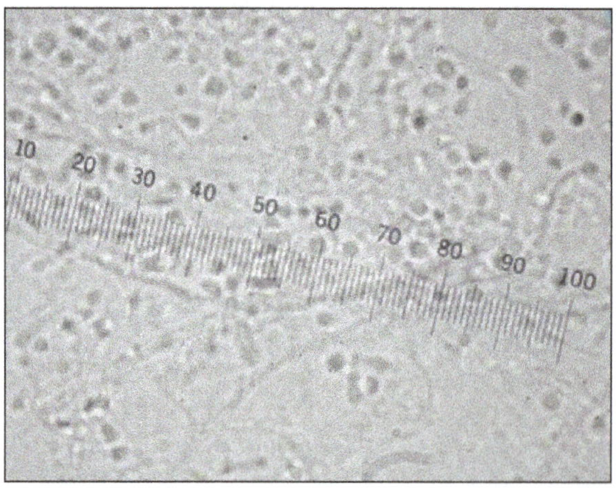

Reproduction in Fungi

Fungi reproduce by asexual, sexual and parasexual means. Asexual reproduction is the commonest mode in most fungi with fungi participating in sexual mode only under certain circumstances. The form of fungus undergoing asexual reproduction is known as anamorph (or imperfect stage) and when the same fungus is undergoing sexual reproduction, the form is said to be teleomorph (or perfect stage). The whole fungus, including both the forms is referred as holomorph.

Asexual Reproduction

Asexual propagules are termed either spores or conidia depending on their mode of production. Asexual spores are produced following mitosis whereas sexual spores are produced following meiosis.

The asexual spores of zygomycetes, which are known as sporangiospores form within sac like structure known as sporangia. The sporangiospores result from the mitotic cleavage of cytoplasm in the sporangium. The sporangia are borne on special hyphae called sporangiophore. This endogenous process of spore formation within a sac is known as sporogenesis.

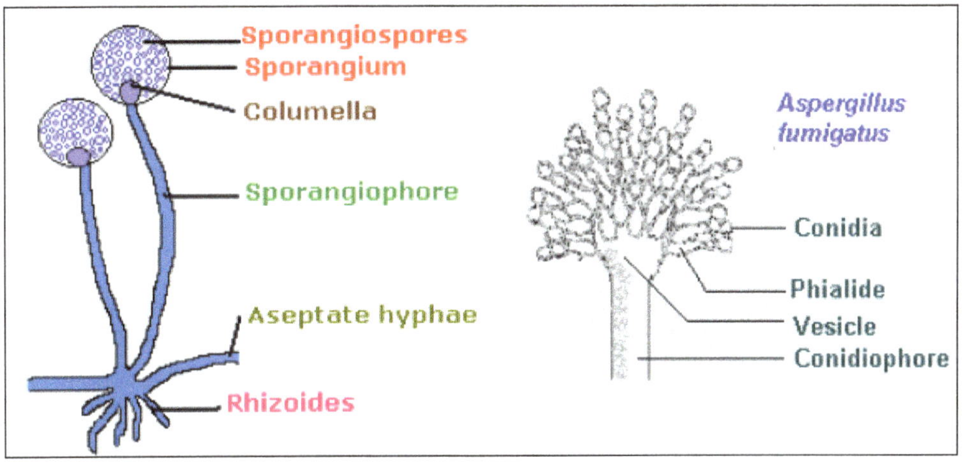

Conidia arise either by budding off conidiogenous hyphae or by differentiation of preformed hyphae. These develop following mitosis of a parent nucleus and are formed in any manner except involving cytoplasmic cleavage. This exogenous process is known as conidiogenesis, a process that occurs both in yeasts and moulds. Conidia are borne on specialised structures called conidiophore.

It is the type of reproduction which involves the somatic portion of the fungal thallus. It occurs by the following methods.

Fragmentation

In this process, the mycelium breaks into two or more similar fragments either accidentally or due to some external force. Each fragment grows into a new mycelium.

Budding

The parent cell produces one or more projections called buds, which later develop necessary structures and detach to grow into new individuals. Budding is common in unicellular forms like yeast.

Fission

In this process, the parent cell splits into two equal halves, each of which develops into a new individual. Fission is also common in yeast.

Sclerotia

In some cases, as in Claviceps, the hyphae become interwoven to form a compact mass and get surrounded by a hard covering or rind. Such structures are called SCLEROTIA. They remain dormant under unfavourable conditions and germinate into new mycelia on the return of favourable conditions.

Rhizomorphs

In some higher fungi, several hyphae may become interwoven to form rope-like structures called rhizomorphs. Under favourable conditions, they resume growth to give rise to new mycelia.

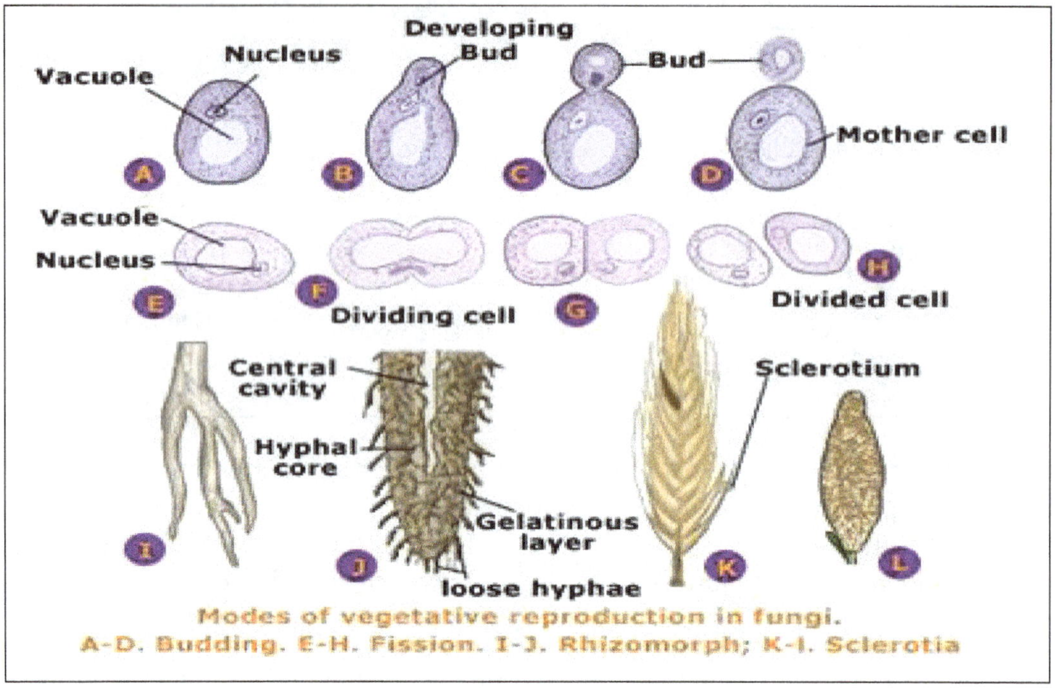

Modes of Vegetative Reproduction.

Asexual Reproductive Structures

It is the types of reproduction in which special reproductive structures called spores or propagates are formed. The fungal spores always result from mitosis and hence are described as mitospores. Following are the types of spores produced in different groups of fungi:

Zoospores

They are flagellated, motile spores produced inside structures called zoosporangia. These spores do not have a cell wall. Such spores are produced in lower fungi such as Achyla and Saprolegnia.

Sporagiospores

These are non-motile spores produced inside structures called sporangia in fungi such as Rhizopus and Mucor. These spores are dispersed by wind.

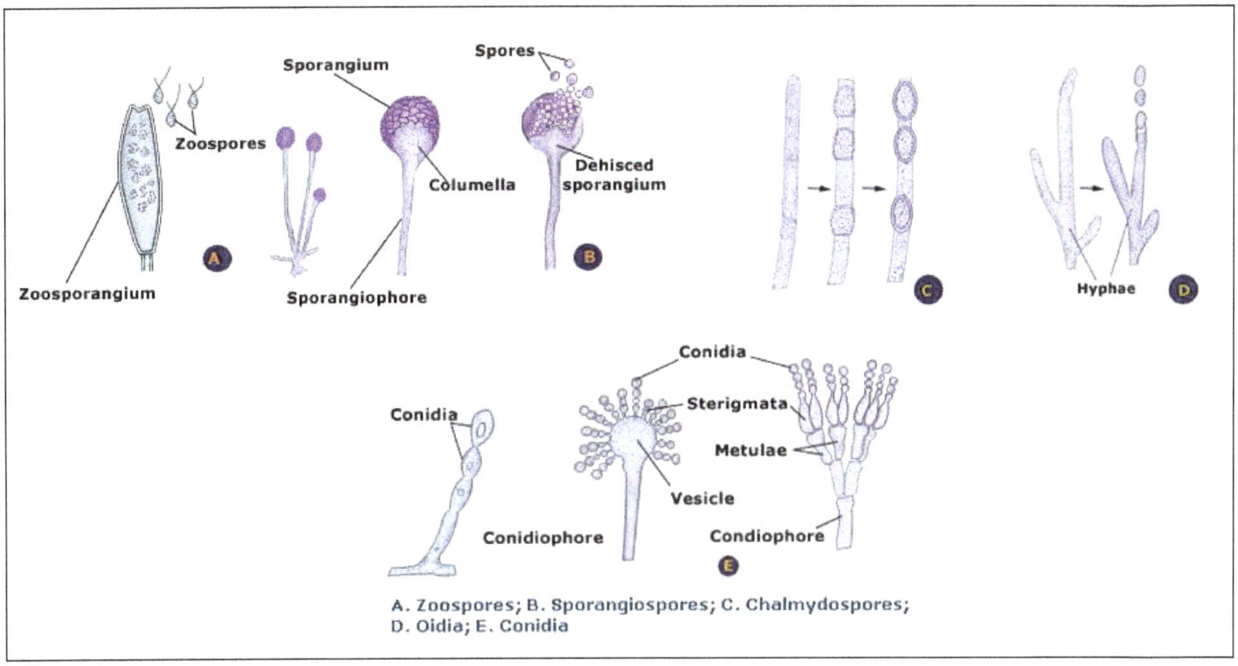

Modes of Asexual Reproduction.

Chlamydospores

These are thick walled resting spores which arise directly from hyphal cells. They store reserve food.

Oidia

These are spore like structures formed by the breaking up of hypha cells. They do not store reserve food and hence cannot survive under unfavourable conditions. Such spores are produced in Rhizopus.

Conidia

These are non-motile spores produced singly or in chains at the tip of the hypha branches that are called conidiophores. Such spores are produced in fungi like Aspergillus and Penicillium.

Sexual Reproduction

Sexual reproduction is known to occur in all groups of fungi except the Fungi imperfecti or Dueteromycetes. It may involve fusion of gametes, gametangia or hyphae. The process may involve only fusion of cytoplasm (plasmogamy) or fusion of nuclei (karyogamy) or production of meiotic spores (meiospores).

In most of the lower fungi plasmogamy is immediately followed by karyogamy and meiosis. In higher fungi karyogamy is often delayed so that the hyphae remain dikaryotic. This phase of fungal life cycle is called dikaryophase. Such fungi complete their life cycle in three phases a haplophase, a dikaryophase and a diplophase.

Sexual fusion in fungi is of different types, as follows:

Planogametic Copulation

Here motile gametes called planogametes undergo fusion. When both the gametes are motile and morphologically similar, the fusion process is called isogamy.

Eg: Synchytrium, when both the gametes are motile but differ in their size, the fusion process is called anisogamy.

Eg: Allomyces, when one gamete (male) is smaller and motile and the other (female) gamete is larger and non-motile, the fusion process is called heterogamy.

Gametangial Contact

Here, gamete bearing structures called gametangia come closer to each other and develop a fertilisation tube through which the male gamete migrates into the female gametangium. Eg: Phytophthora, Albugo.

Gametangial Copulation

Here, the gametangia fuse with each other, lose their identity and develop into a zygospore. Eg.: Mucor, Rhizopus.

Spermatisation

In some fungi like Puccinia, tiny unicellular spore like structures called spermatia are formed.

They get transferred to female gametangia through various agencies.

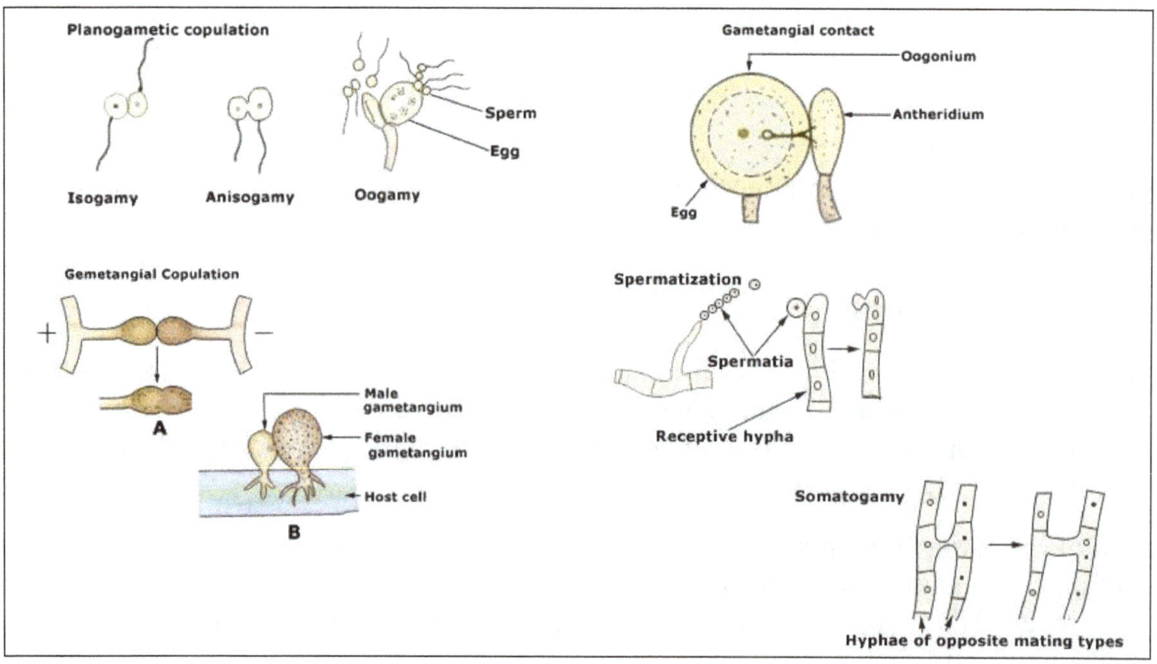

Types of Sexual Reproduction in Fungi.

Somatogamy

In examples like Agaricus, fusion occurs between two somatic cells and involves only plasmogamy. This results in the formation of dikaryotic hyphae. Hence, the process is called dikaryotization.

Homothallism and Heterothallism

Based on the compatibility in sexual reproduction the fungal hyphae can be distinguished into two types homothallic and heterothallic. In homothallic forms, fusion occurs between the genetically similar strains or mating types. In such forms, meiosis results in the formation of genetically identical spores. In the heterothallic forms, fusion occurs between the genetically different mating types or strains. The strains are genetically compatible and are designated as + strain and strain. In such forms meiosis results in the formation of both the strains, in equal numbers. Heterothallism is a device to prevent inbreeding and promote out breeding.

Classification of Fungi

Fungi are eukaryotic microorganisms. They can occur as yeasts, moulds, or as a combination of both forms. Some fungi are capable of causing superficial, cutaneous, subcutaneous, systemic or allergic diseases. Yeasts are microscopic fungi consisting of solitary cells that reproduce by budding. Moulds, in contrast, occur in long filaments known as hyphae, which grow by apical extension. Regardless of their shape or size, fungi are all heterotrophic and digest their food externally by releasing hydrolytic enzymes into their immediate surroundings (absorptive nutrition). Other characteristics of fungi are the ability to synthesize lysine by the L-α-adipic acid biosynthetic pathway and possession of a chitinous cell wall, plasma membranes containing the sterol ergosterol, 80S rRNA, and microtubules composed of tubulin.

- The classification of fungi, like that of bacteria, is designed mainly for practical application but it also bears some relation to phylogenetic considerations.
- The nomenclature is binomial, with a generic and a specific name (eg: Aspergillus niger).
- Species are collected in genera, genera in families (suffix –aceae), families in orders (suffix-ales), and orders in classes (suffix-mycetes).
- The division of mycota, or fungi and moulds, includes the true slime moulds (Myxomycetes), the lower fungi (Phycomycetes), and the higher fungi (Eumycetes).
- Alexopolous and Mims proposed fungal classification in 1979. They place the fungi including the slime molds in the kingdom mycetae of the super kingdom Eukaryota which, in addition, includes four other kingdoms.
- They divide the kingdom mycetae into three divisions namely:
    - Gymnomycota,
    - Mastigomycota and
    - Amastigomycota.

Division I Gymnomycota

- The division is subdivided into subdivision, classes, sub-classes, and orders.
- It includes phagotrophic organism devoid of cell walls.
- This division comprises two subdivisions:
    - Acrasiogymnomycotina and
    - Plasmodiogynomycotina.

Subdivision 1: Acrasiogymnomycotina

It includes a single class Acrasiomycetes.

Class 1: Acrasiomycetes

- Lacks flagellated cells except for one species. The class comprises two subclasses.
- Acrasiomycetidae and Dictyosteliomycetidae.

Subdivision 2: Plasmodiogymnomycotina

It is divided into two classes:

Class 1: Protosteliomycetes

Class 2: Mycomycetes

It includes the true slime mould and comprises three sub classes namely:

Sub Class 1: Ceratiomyxomycomycetidae

Order – Ceratiomyxales

Sub Class 2: Mycogasteomycetidae

It comprises four orders.

Order:

1. Liceales
2. Echinosteleales
3. Trichlales
4. Physarales

Sub Class 3: Stemonitomycetidae

Order 1: Stemonitales

Division II Mastigomycota

Includes fungi with absorptive nutrition, unicellular or filamentous, mycelium coenocytic.

It comprises two sub divisions:

Sub Division 1: Haplomastigomycotina

Includes fungi with uni-or, bi-flagellate zoospores.

Class 1: Chytridiomycetes– Fungi producing zoospores furnished with a single whiplash flagellum inserted at the posterior end.

Class 2: Hyphochytridiomycetes- Motile cells with a single tinsel flagellum inserted at the anterior end.

Class 3: Plasmodiophoromycetes- Parasitic fungi producing biflagellate motile cells with both the flagella of whiplash type inserted at the anterior end.

Sub Division 2: Diplomastigomycotima Sexual Reproduction Ooagamous, Zoospores Biflagellate.

Class 1: Oomycetes

It comprises four orders.

Order:

1. Lagenidiales
2. Saprolegnailes
3. Leptomitales
4. Peronosporales

Division III Amastigomycota

Fungi with absorptive nutrition, motile cells lacking, mycelium aseptate or septate.

This includes four sub divisions:

Sub Division 1: Zygomycotina

Class 1: Zygomycetes – it includes six orders.

Class 2: Trichomycetes – it comprises five orders.

Sub Division 2: Ascomycotina

Fungi usually with a septate mycelium producing haploid ascospores in sac like cells called asci.

Class 1: Ascomycetes - divided into five sub classes:

Sub class 1: Hemiascomycetidae - comprising three orders.

Sub class 2: Plectomycetidae - Five orders

Sub class 3: Hymenoascomycetidae – Ten orders

Sub class 4: Laboulbeniomycetidae – Two orders

Sub class 5: Lowloascomycetidae – five orders

Sub Division 3: Basidiomycotina

Septate mycelium, produces basidiospores, exogenously on various types of basidia.

Class 1: Basidiomycetes: it is split into 3 sub clases:

Sub class 1: Holobasidiomycetidae

Sub class 2: Phragmobasidiomycetidae

Sub class 3: Teliomycetidae

Sub Division 4: Deuteromycotina

It includes imperfect fungi in which sexual stage is unknown. It comprises a single form class.

Form Class Deuteromycetes with three form sub classes namely Blastomycetidae, Coelomycetidae and Hyphomycetidae.

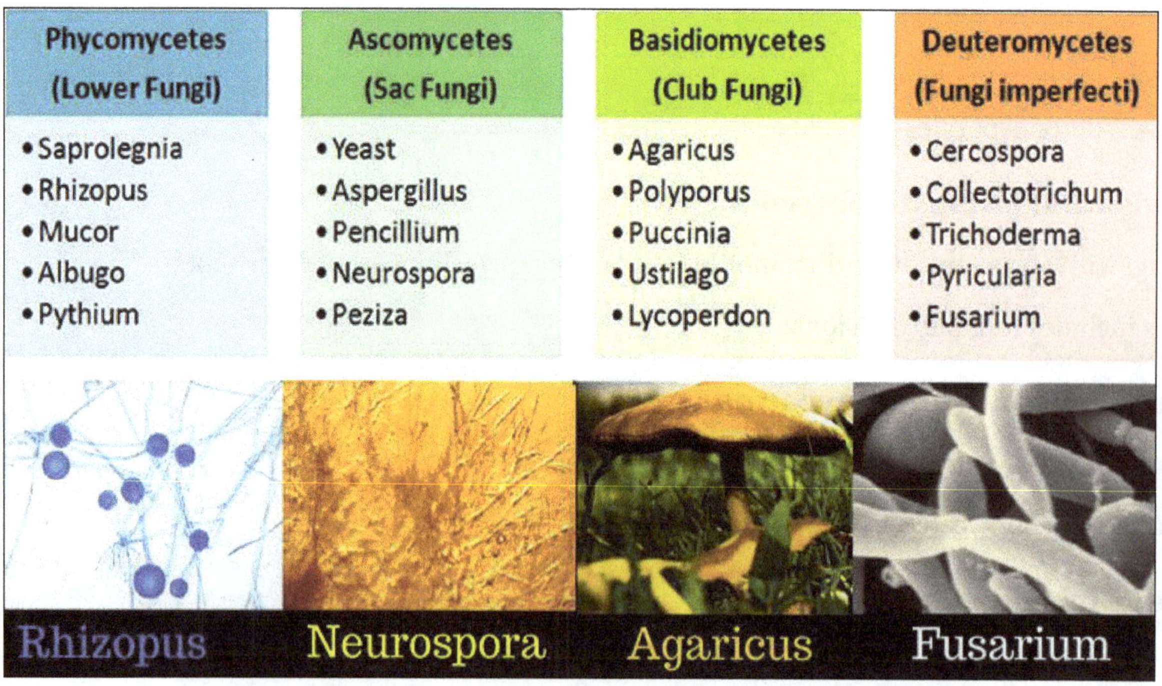

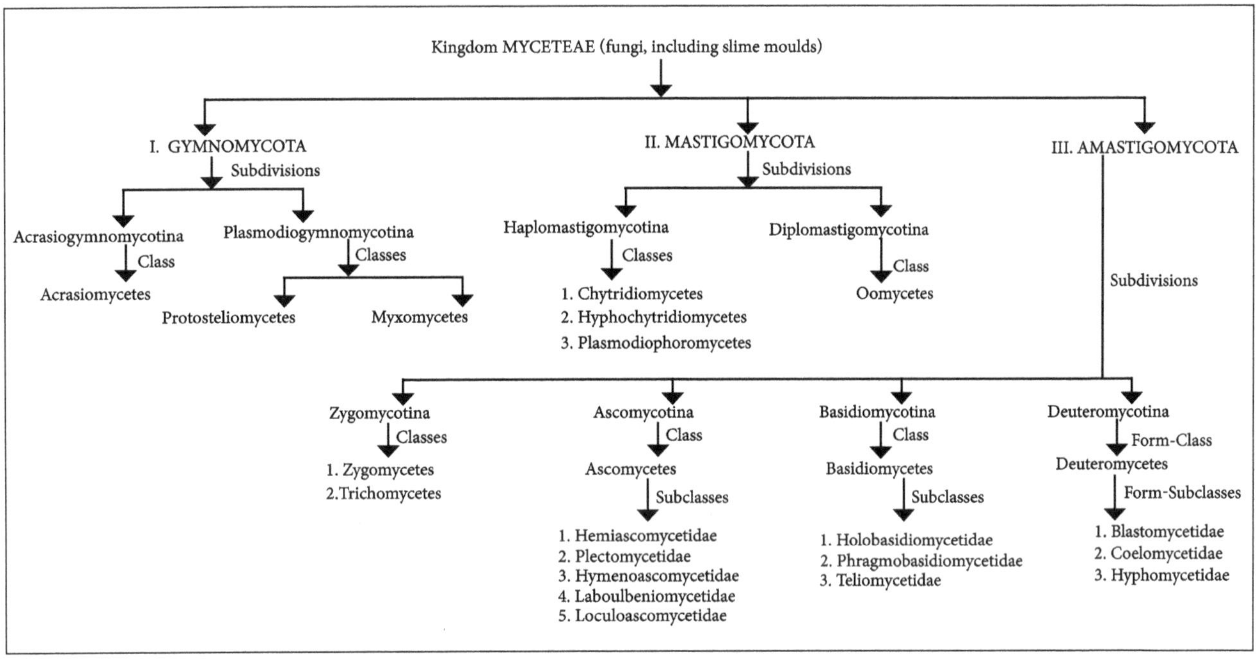

System proposed by Constantine john Alexopoulos and Charles W Mims (1979).

Morphological Classification:

- Moulds-They are hyphae in form Eg. Ringworm or dermatophytes.
- Yeasts-Single cell that bud to reproduce Eg. Cryptococcus Neoformans.
- Yeast Like-Form pseudo hyphae Eg. Candida albicans.
- Dimorphic fungi-fungi having yeast form in tissue and mould in culture Eg. Blastomyces dermatitides.

On the Basis of Spore Production

On the basis of the organisation of the vegetative thallus, the morphology of reproductive structures, the way of spores production and particular life cycle involved the kingdom mycota is classified into following divisions.

Phycomycetes

- It includes the simplest type of fungi. It is also called as Algae-Fungi because most of the characteristics of them are similar to algae like Vaucheria.
- They have simple thallus which is unicellular or coenocytic or aseptate filaments.
- They reproduce asexually by the formation of zoospores or non-motile spores.
- Sexual reproduction is isogamous or heterogamous which takes place by gametangial contact.

- The diploid phase is represented by zygote.
- Phycomycetes has been classified into subclasses: (a) oomycetes and (b) zygomycetes.

Oomycetes

- Oomycetes range from a primitive unicellular thallus to a profusely branched filamentous mycelium.
- Many members of them are terrestrial and obligate parasites.
- Asexually they reproduce by biflagellate zoospores.
- Sexual reproduction is oogamy that involves the fusion of male and female gametes to form oospore.
- Oospore undergoes meioses to produce haploid biflagellate zoospores.
- Example; Phytophthora infestans (causes potato blight).

Zygomycetes

- The group is named zygomycetes because a diploid resting spore called the zygospore is formed during the life cycle.
- They are mostly saprophytic, some others are parasites on plants and animals.
- The vegetative body is mycelium which is well developed, profusely branched and coenocytic.
- The absence of motile sexual or asexual cells.
- The asexual reproduction takes place by sporangiospores, aplanospores or by conidia.
- Sexual reproduction occurs by conjugation of gametangia resulting in the formation of zygospore.
- Examples; Rhizopus, Mucor etc.

Ascomycetes

The species of ascomycetes are called the sac fungi because they produce sexual pores within the sac-like vascus.

General Characteristics:

- Ascomycetes are mostly terrestrial occurring as saprophytes or parasites.
- They have well-developed, branched, septate mycelium except yeast. Yeast is a unicellular fungus.
- Asexually they reproduce by non-motile spores, conidia, oidia or chlamydospores.
- Sexual reproduction takes place by the fusion of gametangia of opposite mating types.

- There is absence of motile cells.
- Examples, Saccharomyces cerevisiae, Penicillium, Aspergillus etc.

Basidiomycetes

- The members of basidiomycetes are saprophytic or parasitic. The group is named basidiomycetes as they produce the basidiospores at the club-shaped basidium during sexual reproduction.
- Mycelium is highly developed, profusely branched and septate.
- The mycelia are differentiated into two mating types; (+ve) and (-ve).
- There are two kinds of mycelium; primary mycelium and secondary mycelium.
- Asexual reproduction takes place by fragmentation, budding, oidia, conidia or chlamydospore.
- The dikaryotic cell is formed during sexual reproduction.
- The absence of motile cell throughout the life cycle.
- Basidiomycetes are the most advanced fungi as their fructifications are often large and prominent.
- Examples; Mushrooms, Puccinia, Ustilago etc.

Deuteromycetes (The Imperfect Fungi)

- Deuteromycetes compromises more than 17000 species of the diverse habits and habitats. It is considered as an artificial class of fungi.
- The fungi are saprophytes as well as parasites. Parasitic fungi cause serious diseases to plants, animals including human beings.
- Some of them are unicellular while others are multicellular.
- They reproduce asexually by conidia along with some other types of spores.
- The sexual reproduction is entirely absent.
- The asexual stage or imperfect stage in Deuteromycetes is well defined. But the sexual or perfect stage is absent in life cycle, therefore, they are called 'Fungi Imperfecti'.
- Example; Alternaria, Fusarium, Helminthosporium etc.

Fungal Pathogenicity

As with the bacteria, fungal virulence factors can be divided into two categories: virulence factors that promote fungal colonization of the host; and virulence factors that damage the host.

Virulence Factors that Promote Fungal Colonization

Virulence factors that promote fungal colonization of the host include the ability to:

- Adhere to host cells and resist physical removal;
- Invade host cells;
- Compete for nutrients;
- Resist innate immune defenses such as phagocytosis and complement; and
- Evade adaptive immune defenses.

Examples of virulence factors that promote fungal colonization include:

1. A compromised immune system is the primary predisposing factor for serious fungal infections. A person highly immunosuppressed, such as a person taking immunosuppressive drugs to suppress transplant rejection, or a person with advancing HIV infection, or a person with other immunosuppressive disorders, becomes very susceptible to infections by fungi generally considered not very harmful to a healthy person with normal defenses.
2. As with bacteria, the ability to adhere to host cells with cell wall adhesins seems to play a role in fungal virulence.
3. Some fungi produce capsules allowing them to resist phagocytic engulfment, such as the yeast *Cryptococcus neoformans* and the yeast form of *Histoplasma capsulatum*.
4. *Candida albicans* stimulates the production of a cytokine called GM-CSF and this cytokine can suppress the production of complement by monocytes and macrophages. This may decrease the production of the opsonin C3b as well as the complement proteins that enhance chemotaxis of phagocytes.
5. *C. albicans* also appears to be able to acquire iron from red blood cells.
6. *C. albicans* produces acid proteases and phospholipases that aid in the penetration and damage of host cell membranes.
7. Some fungi are more resistant to phagocytic destruction, e.g., *Candida albicans, Histoplasma capsulatum*, and *Coccidioides immitis*.
8. There is evidence that when the yeast form of *Candida* enters the blood it activates genes allowing it to switch from its budding form to its hyphal form. In addition, when engulfed by macrophages, it starts producing the tubular germ tubes which penetrate the membrane of the macrophage thus causing its death.

   A movie of *Candida* killing a macrophage from within from the Theriot Lab Website at Stanford University Medical School: *Candida albicans* killing macrophages from inside out.
9. Factors such as body temperature, osmotic stress, oxidative stress, and certain human hor-

mones activate a dimorphism-regulating histidine kinase enzyme in dimorphic molds, such as *Histoplasma capsulatum, Blastomyces dermatitidis,* and *Coccidioides immitis,* causing them to switch from their avirulent mold form to their virulent yeast form. It also triggers the yeast *Candida albicans* to switch from its yeast form to its more virulent hyphal form.

Virulence Factors that Damage the Host

Like bacteria, fungal PAMPs binding to PRRs can trigger excessive cytokine production leading to a harmful inflammatory response that damages tissues and organs. As fungi grow in the body, they can secrete enzymes to digest cells. These include proteases, phospholipases, and elastases. In response to both the fungus and to cell injury, cytokines are released. As seen earlier under Bacterial Pathogenesis, this leads to an inflammatory response and extracellular killing by phagocytes that leads to further destruction of host tissues.

Many molds secrete mycotoxins, especially when growing on grains, nuts and beans. These toxins may cause a variety of effects in humans and animals if ingested including loss of muscle coordination, weight loss, and tremors. Some mycotoxins are mutagenic and carcinogenic. Aflatoxins, produced by certain *Aspergillus* species, are especially carcinogenic. A mold called *Stachybotrys chartarum* is a mycotoxin producer that has been implicated as a potential serious problem in homes and buildings as one of the causes of "sick building syndrome." Mycotoxin symptoms in humans include dermatitis, inflammation of mucous membranes, cough, fever, headache, and fatigue.

Uses of Fungi

There are multiple uses of fungi. Let us study about a few major ones.

Economic importance of fungi: Fungi have both positive and negative roles in our daily life. So they are our friends as well as enemy.

Benefit of Fungi

Directly or indirectly fungi are beneficial to human being. Fungi are used in medicine industry, as food, in food preparation, in other industry and also in agriculture. Some of the useful activities are:

Preparation of Medicine

Different types of fungi are used in the production of important numbers of drugs. The most important species are Penicillium notatum, Claviceps purpurea, Saccharo myces cerevisiae, Aspergillus proliferous etc.

Antibiotics

Antibiotics are the metabolic products of some microorganisms which are active against other microorganism. Wonder drug Penicillin from Penicillium notatum and drug Fusidin (Fusidic acid) from Fusidium coccineum.

Name of antibiotics	Produced fungi	Range of activity
1. Penicillin	Pencillium notatum and P. crysogenum	Bacteria (both Gram + and –)
2. Griseofulvin	P. nigricans P. griseofulvum	Fungi
3. Cephalosporin	Acremonium sp.	Bacteria (Gram +)
4. Citrinin	P. citrinum	Fungi
5. Palutin	P. palutum	Fungi and Bacteria
6. Fumagillin	Aspergillus fumigatus	Protozoa
7. Fusidic acid	Fusidium coccineum	Bacteria
8. Viridin	Tichoderma viridi	Fungi

Vitamins

Vitamins are the micronutrients required for the growth of living organisms. Vitamin B-complex, Vitamin A and Vitamin B-12 are found respectively from Saccharomyces cerevisiae, and Eremothemium ashbyii.

Steroid

Rheumatic arthritis, allergy and some other diseases are controlled by steroid. Many fungi have the capacity to synthesize different steroids. Steroid like cortisone is produced by Aspergillus niger from plant glycosides by fermentation.

Alkaloid

Several alkaloids are produced and accumulated in the sclerotium of Claviceps purpurea which causes Ergot disease of rye. Out of several alkaloids, Ergo- metrine and its semisynthetic analogues like methyl ergometrine and methyl ergometrine maleate have notable uterine action; those control haemorrhage of mother during child's birth, having side- effect with increase in blood pressure and decreased milk secretion.

Foods

Fungi are used as food by humans from a long time ago. Some fungi have been used directly as food and some are used in food processing:

Direct Use

Fruit bodies of some fungi, like Mushroom and truffles are used as food due to their high protein content (21-30% on dry weight) and have good amount of lysine, an amino acid; minerals like Na, Ca, K and P; Vitamins like B, C, D and K and very little amount of fat.

These are recommended as ideal foods for heart patients and diabetes. The above-mentioned fungi can grow artificially at the commercial level. Mushroom cultivation has recently gained considerable popularity and has contributed to the national economy in some East Asian countries.

Fungi in Industry

Many fungi are used in the production of alcohol, bread, cheese, enzyme and organic acids.

Alcohol Production

Alcoholic fermentation by fungi is the basis of brewing industry. The enzyme zymase of microorganisms like yeast is responsible for alcohol production.

Wines are produced from grapes or other fruits by Saccharomyces ellipsoideus with about 14% alcohol concentration. Beer is brewed from barley malt by Saccharomyces cerevisiae with 3-8% alcohol production.

Bread and Cake Production

During alcoholic fermentation by yeast, CO_2 being released as bubbles are used in baking industry to make the breads and cakes as spongy in appearance.

Cheese Production

Some species of Penicillium (P. roquiforti and P. camemberti) are used in the produc¬tion of Roquefort and Camembert cheese by hydrolysis of fats and also to develop specific flavour to cheese.

Enzyme and Organic Acid Production

Many fungi are used in the commercial production of enzymes and different organic acids.

List of some fungi along with produced enzymes and/or acids and their uses are given:

Enzyme Organic acid	Produced fungi	Uses
Enzymes		
1. Amylase	Aspergillus oryzae. A. niger	Alcohol industry and in pharmaceuticals.
2. Cellulase	Trichoderma reesli	Production of cheese and hydrolysis of cellulose
3. Invertase	Saccharomyces Cerevisiae	Paper industry and confectionary
4. Zymase	Saccharomyces cerevisiae	Ethyle alcohol production
Organic acids		
1. Citric acid	Aspergillus niger, A. wentil	Soft drinks and other food. Manufacture of ink and leather tanning
2. Fumaric acid	Rhizopus stolonifier	Manufacture of wetting agents
3. Gallic acid	Aspergillus gallomyces, Penicillum glaucum	Manufacture of ink and dyes

4. Gluconic acid	Aspergillus niger, Penicillium Purpurogenum	In textile, leather, food and photographic industries and also in pharmaceuticals.
5. Kojic acid	Aspergillus oryzae	As insecticide and antibiotic
6. Itaconic acid	Aspergillus terreus, A. itaconicum	Manufacture of synthetic fibre and plasticisers

Soil Fertility

Decomposition of litter and wood, mainly in the forest, takes place by the combined action of different type of fungi. Fungi like Fusarium, Chaetomium, Chitridium, Penicillium, Aspergillus etc., can decompose the structural polymers such as cellulose, hemicellulose, lipid, protein, starch etc.

By decomposing the organic matters, fungi help to increase minerals and other substances, thereby the fertility of soil is increased.

Plant Nutrition

Several fungal members like Rhizoctonia, Tricholoma, Boletus, Phallus, Amanita etc., associated with the roots of higher plants form mycorrhizal relationship. The fungal partner supplies water and minerals and in turn, they take nutrition from the plant.

As Insecticide: Fungi like Cordyceps melonthae, are used as insecticides to control different types of insects.

Biological Research

Fungi like Neurospora, Yeast etc., have been used in genetical and cytological studies. Physarum polysephalum has been used to study DNA-synthesis.

Test Organism

Some strains of Aspergillus niger have been used to detect trace elements like Zn, Cu, and Mo, even if the substances are present in very minute quantity in the substrate. These elements when absorbed by the fungus give a particular colour to the conidia. Similarly, Neurospora crassa has been used to detect Vitamin B complex.

Production Plant Hormone

Some fungi are used to produce plant hormone like Gibberellin by soil fungus Gibberella fujikuroi.

Biological Control

The antagonistic activity of some fungi like Trichoderma sp. showed that it is parasitic on many soil-borne and foliage pathogens. Trichoderma sp. is being used to control plant diseases in sustainable diseases management systems.

Fungal Nutrition and Cellular Biosynthesis

Like animals, fungi are heterotrophs: They use complex organic compounds as a source of carbon rather than fixing carbon dioxide from the atmosphere, as some bacteria and most plants do. In addition, fungi do not fix nitrogen from the atmosphere. Like animals, they must obtain it from their diet. However, unlike most animals that ingest food and then digest it internally in specialized organs, fungi perform these steps in the reverse order. Digestion precedes ingestion. First, exoenzymes, enzymes that catalyze reactions on compounds outside of the cell, are transported out of the hyphae where they break down nutrients in the environment. Then, the smaller molecules produced by the external digestion are absorbed through the large surface areas of the mycelium. As with animal cells, the fungal storage polysaccharide is glycogen rather than starch, as found in plants.

Fungi are mostly saprobes, organisms that derive nutrients from decaying organic matter. They obtain their nutrients from dead or decomposing organic matter, mainly plant material. Fungal exoenzymes are able to break down insoluble polysaccharides, such as the cellulose and lignin of dead wood, into readily absorbable glucose molecules. Decomposers are important components of ecosystems, because they return nutrients locked in dead bodies to a form that is usable for other organisms. This role is discussed in more detail later. Because of their varied metabolic pathways, fungi fulfill an important ecological role and are being investigated as potential tools in bioremediation. For example, some species of fungi can be used to break down diesel oil and polycyclic aromatic hydrocarbons. Other species take up heavy metals such as cadmium and lead.

Like plants, Fungi do not require Carbon dioxide and light as a source of Carbon for their food. The Fungi get attached to the organic matter and absorb Carbohydrates. It absorbs and metabolizes various soluble Carbohydrates like Glucose, Fructose, Xylose, and Sucrose. Also, Fungi have the ability to absorb and process insoluble carbohydrates like cellulose, hemicellulose, and starches along with complex hydrocarbons such as lignin. Many Fungi even absorb Proteins as a source of carbon and nitrogen. Fungi will produce digestive enzymes to polymers extracellular; this helps to utilize insoluble carbohydrates and Proteins. Using the biological catalysts, an enzyme secreted on the surface of the Fungi starts to secure its food. The digestive enzyme helps to break down the food and the root-like substance present of the Fungi called hyphal walls absorbs the food. Food in the form of liquid can only enter into hyphae, the entire mycelial surface of Fungus has the capability to absorb water and minerals entered through hyphae. This is how Fungi obtain their food. For example, The surface of the rotten fruits became soft. This is because of fungal enzymes. Many parasitic Fungi have some specialized features like absorptive organs. This is known as haustoria.

Fungi are broadly classified into three types, based on how Fungi obtain their food.

Types of Nutrition in Fungi

- Saprotrophic Fungi - Fungi obtain food from dead and decayed materials.
- Parasitic Fungi - Get feed from living Organisms and destroy them.
- Symbiotic Fungi - Grow in a living Organism and get mutually benefited.

Saprotrophic Fungi

Like bacteria, saprotrophic Fungi have a huge responsibility to decompose the organic matter in the earth. The saprotrophic Fungi takes responsible for decaying and decomposing the foodstuffs. Many saprotrophs have the ability to destructure and destroy giant structures like timber using the digestive enzyme mycelia. The tropical region's humidity and temperature support the growth of Fungi. The nutritional availability takes responsibility to determine the growth of saprotrophs.

Each Fungus synthesizes the enzyme with different chemical composition. But all Fungi have the same morphological characteristics in culture media. Required carbon is supplied to the Fungi in the form of sugars or starch. Most Fungi absorb the sugar in the form of fructose, maltose, mannose, fructose, and in some least cases sucrose. For a nitrogen source, Fungi compose proteins and produce proteoses, amino acids, and peptones. Some Fungi absorb ammonium compounds and nitrates as a nutrient source. Also, Fungi have the ability to combine and fix atmospheric nitrogen using suitable compounds. To vigorous the growth of Fungi some chemical components like phosphorus, sulfur, magnesium, potassium, manganese, iron, zinc, copper are essential. Also, the least amount of calcium, molybdenum, and gallium are required for species growth.

Fungi require oxygen and hydrogen, which will absorb in the form of water. Also, Fungi require vitamins and minerals like thiamine and biotin to boost the growth of Fungi and reproduction. As Fungi are aerobic Organisms, they require free oxygen for their survival. During its anaerobic condition, it undergoes a fermentation process. Many industries are using saprotrophic Fungi for their fermentation process.

For example, the most known saprotrophic Fungi, which undergo an anaerobic process are Neocallimastix. This can act upon the plant cell wall components such as Xylem and cellulose. But it cannot act on the animal cell walls.

Parasitic Fungi

Parasitic Fungi use to live on living Organisms by invading them. These types of Fungi start extracting Nutrients from the living cytoplasm. This causes disease and death to the host. Most pathogenic fungi are parasites of plants, which enter into the body through the natural opening present in plants like stoma, lenticel in a stem, and broken plants. This causes great damage to the crops. The spores of a pathogenic Fungus fall on the leaves and stems of plants and increase infection of a plant. The tube grows on the surface of the host and absorbs food for Fungi, this invades the tissues and cell walls.

Parasitic Fungi in Humans

Many pathogenic Fungi cause disease in human beings and animals. The parasitic Fungi generally enter the body through a wound in the epidermis. This may enter through insects. For example, parasitic Fungi Claviceps purpurea causes ergotism in human beings. This disease is widely spread among middle-aged people in northern Europe. Other fungal diseases that affect humans are ringworm, aspergillosis, coccidioidomycosis, histoplasmosis, and athlete's foot. People infected by HIV are mainly due to agent acquired immunodeficiency syndrome (AIDS) weakens the immune system. This is mainly due to the parasitic Fungi called Aspergillus fumigatus.

Symbiotic Fungi

The Fungi grows in the other Organism and it does not cause any harmful effects for the living Organism. Here, both the living Organism and Fungi get mutually benefited. The symbiotic Fungi are of two types. They are mycorrhizae and lichen.

Mycorrhiza shows the mutual relationship between the Fungus and plants. This Fungus grows on the root of plants. The Fungus avails its food from the soil and takes shelter from the plants. Likewise, plants utilize the mycelia of Fungi to absorb Nutrients and water.

Lichen shows the mutual relationship between Fungus and photosynthetic Organisms. These Fungi grow in green alga or plants. Here Fungus gets food from photosynthesizers meanwhile photosynthesizers avail essential Nutrients from Fungi, This method explains the nutrition in Fungi.

Predation

Predation is a mode of nutrition for the amoeba. It is very much similar to the mushroom mode of nutrition. Predation catches the microOrganism from the atmosphere through hyphae present in the Fungi and synthesizes the enzyme to break down the cell wall of the Organism and extracts all necessary Nutrients from it. This is how Fungi obtain their food.

Chapter 2

Fungal Infections: An Overview

Fungal Infections

Fungal infection, also known as mycosis, is a disease caused by fungi. Different types are traditionally divided according to the part of the body affected; superficial, subcutaneous, and systemic. Superficial fungal infections include common tinea of the skin, such as tinea of the body, groin, hands, feet and beard, and yeast infections such as pityriasis versicolor. Subcutaneous types include eumycetoma and chromoblastomycosis, which generally affect tissues in and beneath the skin. Systemic fungal infections are more serious and include cryptococcosis, histoplasmosis, pneumocystis pneumonia, aspergillosis and mucormycosis. Signs and symptoms range widely. There is usually a rash with superficial infection. Fungal infection within the skin or under the skin may present with a lump and skin changes. Pneumonia-like symptoms or meningitis may occur with a deeper or systemic infection.

Fungi are everywhere, but only some cause disease. Fungal infection occurs after spores are either breathed in, come into contact with skin or enter the body through the skin such as via a cut, wound or injection. It is more likely to occur in people with a weak immune system. This includes people with illnesses such as HIV/AIDS, and people taking medicines such as steroids or cancer treatments. Fungi that cause infections in people include yeasts, molds and fungi that are able to exist as both a mold and yeast. The yeast *Candida albicans* can live in people without producing symptoms, and is able to cause both superficial mild candidiasis in healthy people, such as oral thrush or vaginal yeast infection, and severe systemic candidiasis in those who cannot fight infection themselves.

Diagnosis is generally based on signs and symptoms, microscopy, culture, sometimes requiring a biopsy and the aid of medical imaging. Some superficial fungal infections of the skin can appear similar to other skin conditions such as eczema and lichen planus. Treatment is generally performed using antifungal medicines, usually in the form of a cream or by mouth or injection, depending on the specific infection and its extent. Some require surgically cutting out infected tissue.

Fungal infections have a world-wide distribution and are common, affecting more than one billion people every year. An estimated 1.7 million deaths from fungal disease were reported in 2020. Several, including sporotrichosis, chromoblastomycosis and mycetoma are neglected.

A wide range of fungal infections occur in other animals, and some can be transmitted from animals to people.

Mycoses are caused by certain fungi; yeasts, molds and some fungi that can exist as both a mold and yeast. They are everywhere and infection occurs after spores are either breathed in, come into contact with skin or enter the body through the skin such as via a cut, wound or injection. *Candida albicans* is the most common cause of fungal infection in people, particularly as oral or vaginal thrush, often following taking antibiotics.

Risk Factors

Fungal infections are more likely in people with weak immune systems. This includes people with illnesses such as HIV/AIDS, and people taking medicines such as steroids or cancer treatments. People with diabetes also tend to develop fungal infections. Very young and very old people, also, are groups at risk.

Individuals being treated with antibiotics are at higher risk of fungal infections.

Children whose immune systems are not functioning properly (such as children with cancer) are at risk of invasive fungal infections.

COVID-19

During the COVID-19 pandemic some fungal infections have been associated with COVID-19. Fungal infections can mimic COVID-19, occur at the same time as COVID-19 and more serious fungal infections can complicate COVID-19. A fungal infection may occur after antibiotics for a bacterial infection which has occurred following COVID-19. The most common serious fungal infections in people with COVID-19 include *aspergillosis* and invasive candidiasis. COVID-19 associated mucormycosis is generally less common, but in 2021 was noted to be significantly more prevalent in India.

Predisposing Factors

Use of drugs that suppress the immune system:

- Cancer chemotherapy drugs.
- Corticosteroids.
- Drugs to prevent rejection of an organ transplant, such as azathioprine, methotrexate, and cyclosporine.
- Tumor necrosis factor inhibitors (used to treat rheumatoid arthritis and related disorders).

Candida infections arise due to alteration in host defense system where both immunological and non-immunological factors play crucial roles making the conditions favorable for proliferation of Candida.

Immunological Factors

The following section describes the immunological predisposing factor which contributes to enhanced susceptibility to candidal infections.

HIV/AIDS

According to the Joint United Nations Programme (2009) on HIV/AIDS and the National AIDS Control Organization (2008), there is an estimation of 2.4 million cases of HIV infection worldwide and 22.7 per 100,000 in India respectively. The immunocompromised or HIV infected patients are more prone to oral and pharyngeal candidiasis. It has been estimated that more than 90% of HIV patients suffer from fungal infections during the progression of disease. The prevalence of candidal infections all over the world is 18%. It has been found that HIV patients suffering from cutaneous candidiasis have low $CD4^+$ lymphocyte count and elevation in RNA load. Other than regular virulence factors in Candida necessary for pathogenesis such as secreted aspartyl proteases are also important for the same but its activity depends on host conditions. Role of Natural killer cells (NK) in immune system against pathogens is well known. They work as immune effectors that directly bind to pathogen and kill them through perforin dependent mechanisms. The cascade involves the receptor NKp30 receptor which is required for fungi and cell conjugate formation, phosphatidylinositol 3-kinase (PI3K) signaling and perforin release. But in case of HIV patients, NKp30 receptors have low activity which accounts for defective antifungal activity of NK cells. Among the fungal pathogens, it has been found that *C. albicans* is the most prevalent species (68.5%) followed by *C. tropicalis* (7.4%), *C. krusei* (6.4%), *C. parapsilosis* (3.0%) and C. sake (2.5%). In HIV infected candidiasis patients, a Th17 functional subset of T helper cells is an important asset which is guarding against this fungus. The selective loss of T helper cells along with the progression of HIV infection causes the decay of fungal containment on the oral epithelium which in turn allows *C. albicans* to express its pathogenic potential. Recent studies have shown that *C. albicans* inhibits the replication of HIV-1 in macrophages and dendritic cells. The inhibition is also contributed by host restriction factors which are able to block retroviral replication. The main cytidine deaminases are APOBEC3G and APOBEC3F that introduces G to A substitutions in the HIV-1 genome which inhibits viral replication. This can be used in antiretroviral therapy but the mucocutaneous candidiasis is also prevalent in HIV patients.

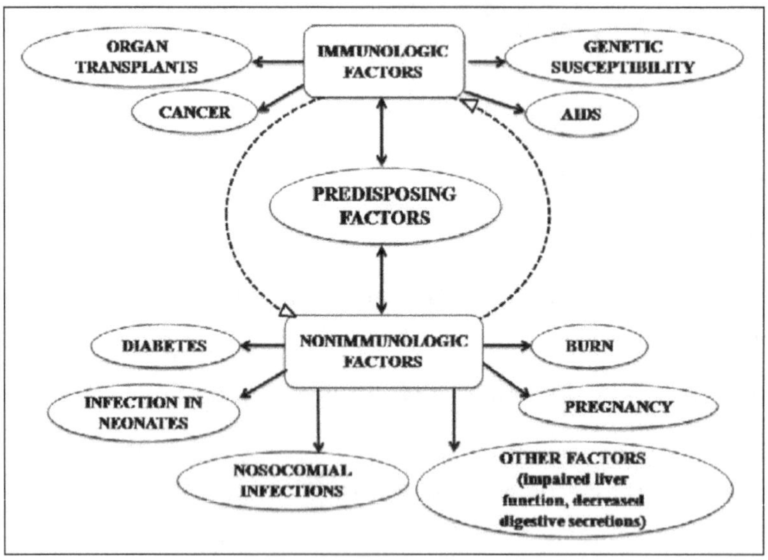

Predisposing factors leading to Candida infections.

The study on correlation between $CD4^+$ counts and the prevalence of candidiasis suggests that $CD4^+$ lymphocyte counts to be a marker of HIV disease progression. The introduction of anti-human immunodeficiency virus drugs of the aspartic protease inhibitor-type (HIV PIs) can be used as a potent agent for inhibition of secretion of aspartic proteases (saps) which is a virulence factor in *C. albicans*. These enzymes can degrade critical host defense components like complement and epithelial defensive proteins such as histatin-5 and E-cadherin. The two subunit vaccines which are based on antigens dominantly expressed by *C. albicans* in vivo are Als3 adhesin and Sap2 which have been recently undergone phase 1 clinical trial. But much new insights are needed in order to combat the fungal infections during this immunocompromised condition.

Organ Transplant

The fungal infections are predominantly prevailing in cases of organ transplantation. It has been reported that fungal infections are the second most common cause of mortality in kidney transplants due to immunosuppressive status of the patients. In organ transplantation, in order to prevent graft rejection, certain drugs are given to the patients as a part of immunosuppressive therapy to suppress the host immune status. The action of these drugs reduces the natural immune response resulting in increased susceptibility to fungal infections and particularly opportunistic organism like *C. albicans*. The prevalence of candidiasis in organ transplants is 7%. Mostly in case of renal transplantation, Candida can become more prevalent after organ transplantation and can lead to more severe infections in bloodstream leading to candidemia. The most frequent form of oral candidiasis in renal transplantation patients is denture stomatitis which is followed by angular chelitis and pseudomembraneous candidiasis. The chances of severe candidiasis increases after immediate post-transplantation period. Invasive fungal infections are the most common causes of mortality in cases of renal transplantation and associated with parenteral nutrition, abdominal surgery and broad spectrum antibiotic therapy. The most prevalent species of Candida is *C. albicans* (86.4%) as reported in a case study of kidney transplants in Brazil. In case of liver transplantation, the prevalence of *Candida* species are *C. albicans* (50%), *C. glabrata* (12.5%), *C. parapsilosis* (12.5%), *C. krusei* (12.5%), *C. lusitaniae* (6.2%), *C. tropicalis* (6.2%) and multiple others (25%). The predisposing factors to fungal infection in patients of lung transplantation includes: preoperative chronic lung diseases and inherent palliative immunosuppression, intraoperative complications such as abnormalities in the bronchial anastomosis or lung injury, and postoperative complications such as enhanced immunosuppression for early rejection, graft dysfunction, concurrent viral and bacterial infections, and bronchiolitis obliterans syndrome.

Cancer

Candida is being ranked among the ten prominent pathogen affecting leukemia patients, resulting in 25-60% mortality rates. In blood tumors, candidemia caused by the *Candida* species affecting the patients are *C. albicans* (33%), *C. guilliermondii* (26%), *C. parapsilosis* (12%), *C. krusei* (8%), *C. lusitaniae* (5%), *C. famata* (4%), *C. tropicalis* (4%), *C. glabrata* (4%), and *C. pelliculosa* (4%). The incidence of candidiasis in cancer patients is around 43.2%. Cancer and chemotherapy results in immunosuppression which gives opportunity for emergence of fungal infection. The outcome is the cellular and humoral immune dysfunction and mucosal damage due to chemotherapy in ovarian and lung cancer. In a study, it has been observed that there is a deficiency of MPO (myeloperoxidase) which is an important risk factor for invasive candidiasis. The decreased level of TNF-α (Tumour Necrosis Factor) is also the result of *Candida* invasion only. MMPs (matrix metalloproteinases) are involved in degradation of extracellular matrix and tumour cell evasion which leads to metastasis in cancer. The MMP2, 3, and 9 increases in breast cancer as they are involved in invasion, metastasis and tumor angiogenesis. The breast cancer patients are susceptible to candidiasis and there is a positive effect of candidiasis on the metastasis and tumor progression in breast cancer patients. It has been found that *Candida* is involved in cell cycle arrest and blocks the proliferation of host cells, PGE2 (Prostaglandin E2) synthase expression (involved in eicosanoid and glutathione metabolism) and thus PGE2 production in patients suffering from HPV (human papillomavirus) 16 virus infections. Interleukin is known to play a key role in mammalian immune system. The cancer patients who have deficient IL-17 receptor or low secretion of IL17 are highly susceptible to systemic candidiasis. More often, candidiasis is a common side effect of chemotherapy for malignant cancer. It has been found that thrombospondin-1 (extracellular matrix protein which is released at tissue injury sites) enhances the pathogenesis of disseminated candidiasis by creating an imbalance in the host immune response which leads to impaired fungal clearance, reduced phagocytic function and increased mortality.

Secreted aspartyl proteinase 2 (Sap2) is a virulence related trait of *Candida* and patients suffering from candidiasis have high titre values of Sap2. The candidiasis does not have significant clinical symptoms and hence its diagnostic methods have less sensitivity. For diagnostic purposes, Sap2 found in serum samples of cancer patients can be used for detection of *Candida* by an indirect competitive enzyme linked immunosorbent assay. The antifungal drug echinocandin was used as a first line drug in candidemia affecting blood tumor patients. Caspofungin and voriconazole drugs have shown immunomodulatory effect on human peripheral blood mononuclear cells (PBMC). The interaction between the drug and cells results in Th1-type cytokine secretion which assists in removal of fungal pathogen.

Genetic Susceptibility

It has been believed that genetic factors must play an important role in determining the susceptibility to *Candida* infections. Mutations in single genes were found to be responsible for severe *Candida* infections in several primary immunodeficiencies that display the clinical picture of monogenetic disorders. The incidence of genetic susceptibility to candidal infections is 8.2%. The monogenetic disorder where CARD 9 gene codes for a protein Dectin-1, if there is a homozygous mutation then it can give rise to increased susceptibility to both mucosal and invasive Candida infections. The other monogenetic disorder that results in an important primary immunodeficiency associated with Candida infections is CMC (chronic mucocutaneous candidiasis). The main cause of autosomal dominant CMC is the mutations in the CC domain of STAT 1 which is a signaling molecule of the type 1 and type 2 IFN-receptor. Several mutations have been found in STAT3 a signaling molecule of the IL-23 receptor, which results in reduced IL-17 production. The mutations in genes coding for cytokines and their receptors have been described to be associated with Candida infections as in IL12Rb1 deficiency which has been linked to mucocutaneous *Candida* infections and found to have increased susceptibility for invasive candidiasis. Genetic variation in Toll like Receptors has also been associated with an increased susceptibility to fungal infections. Three single nucleotide polymorphisms (SNPs) in the TLR1 gene have been shown to influence susceptibility to candidemia. It has been found that although there is a moderate effect on modulation of proinflammatory cytokine production, there is a minor impact of genetic variation in the autophagy genes ATG16L1 (autophagy related 16-like 1) and IRGM (immunity-related GTPase family, M) on the susceptibility to both mucosal and systemic Candida infections. Several studies have been published showing a link between genetic variation and an increased risk for Candida infections, with different genetic pattern between mucosal and systemic candidiasis. So, it can be concluded that the balance between pro- and anti-inflammatory cytokines represent an important component of host defense against both mucosal and systemic candidiasis.

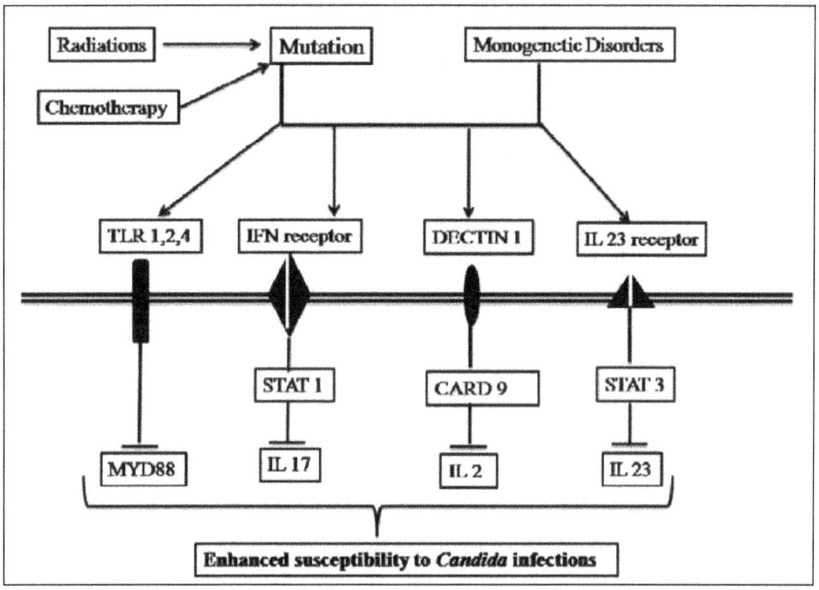

An overview showing the genetic susceptibility to Candida infections due to mutation and monogenetic disorders.

The mutations in TLR (Toll-Like Receptors), IFN (Interferon) receptor, IL (Interleukin) receptor, CARD9 (caspase recruitment domain 9), STAT (Signal transducer and activator of transcription), MYD88 (Myeloid differentiation primary response gene 88) leads to changes in cascade which enhances the susceptibility to Candida infections.

Non-Immunological Factors

The following section describes the non-immunological predisposing factors which contribute to enhanced susceptibility to candidal infections.

Nosocomial Infections

Nowadays, intensive care units (ICU) have emerged as epicenters for candidal infections. The incidence of candidiasis due to nosocomial infections or more commonly referred as hospital acquired infections is 59.7%. Secondary infections in sepsis are caused by *Candida* and candidiasis is the third most reason of blood infections in ICU in hospitals which results into 30-40% mortality rates.

As a matter of fact, widespread and prolonged usage of antifungals has led to the emergence of MDR in *C. albicans*. In a statistical study conducted in ICU in India, the incidence of candidemia was evaluated which clearly shows that the underlying reason for higher risk to candidemia is the use of broad spectrum antibiotics. The patients were given broad spectrum antibiotics and antifungals which resulted in antifungal resistance in turn giving more opportunity for candidal growth. The increased dose of drugs and antibiotics favors the overgrowth of *Candida* and other microbes leading to emergence of MDR strains. Some drugs like ranitidine which are prescribed to patients suffering from ulcers in hospitals often favors the growth of *Candida* and patients become more susceptible to *Candida* infections in hospitals. Thus reduction in antibiotic dosage could be one of the alternative ways to minimize *Candida* infections.

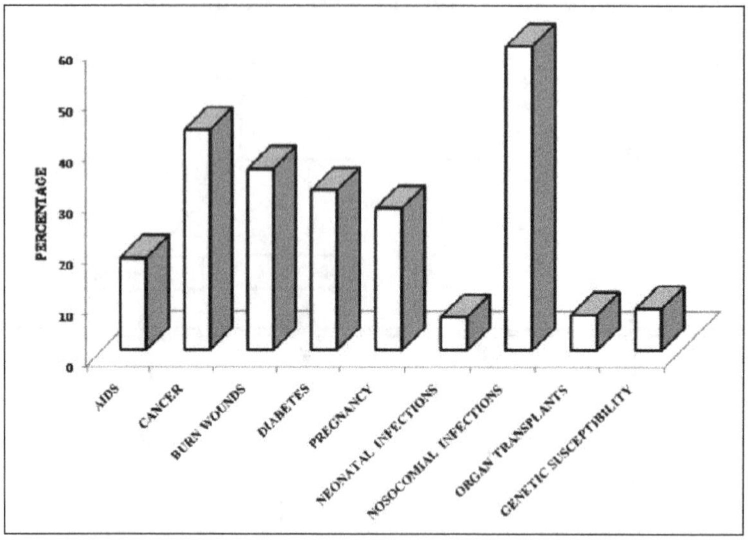

Bar graph showing the contribution of various predisposing factors (expressed as percentage) leading to Candida infections.

The types of *Candida* infections are urinary tract infection, candidemia, surgical site infection and intra-abdominal infection. There is an incidence of invasive candidiasis in neonates in neonatal ICU which results into mortality of low birth weight infants. The underlying cause of candidal infections in neonatal ICU is the horizontal transmission of Candida colony from the newly born who had acquired congenitally and then transmitting to other neonates. In invasive fungal infections in neonates, the predominant causes in ICU are third generation cephalosporin use, neutropenia in first week of life, abdominal surgery, central venous catheter insertion or incubation more than 6 days. Persistent candidemia is the outcome of poor clinical facilities, drug resistance and host related factors on invasive fungal infection in neonatal ICU. It has been studied that patients who have prior abdominal surgery and suffering from chronic PPI (proton pump inhibitor) are predisposed to *Candida* associated intra-abdominal infections. Candidemia is considered as a prevalent factor in noscomial infections. The major causes are ileus, use of proton pump inhibitors, gastrointestinal bleeding, previous stay in the ICU, blood transfusion, vasopressors, requirement for antibiotics, and invasive medical procedures and it can also result in sepsis. The risk factors for mortality are different in early onset candidemia (EOC) and late onset candidemia (LOC). However there is need of improvement in diagnosis and treatment in early infections. The use of catheters in hospitals is one of the causes of urinary tract infection (UTI) in ICU.

Candida species are well known for forming antibiotic resistant biofilms on medical equipment which is one of the major concerns of nosocomial infections. The use of catheters or intravenous devices is a good source for dissemination of biofilm forming fungi. The biofilms are formed on indwelling devices in polymeric matrix and are resistant to the antifungal agents which in turn increase more infection. The biofilms growing on devices like catheters provide a high risk for systemic *candida* infections as they provide entry site to *Candida* directly into patients where they can flourish well. Due to complex structure, they can easily resist the effect of conventional antifungal drugs like amphotericin B and fluconazole.

The bacterial infections may also play as a predisposing factor for candidal infections. The Clostridium difficile infection (CDI) in patients in hospitals is a risk factor for development of candidemia and CDI may predispose for the translocation of Candida. The KPC-producing Klebsiella pneumoniae (KPC-Kp) colonization or infection is also associated with candidemia in hospital acquired infections. Thus the gastrointestinal tube plays as key role in dissemination of Multi Drug Resistant (MDR) microorganisms like *C. difficile* and *K. pneumoniae* and also reservoir for *Candida*. One of the ways to lessen the candida colonization in patients undergoing extensive abdominal surgery is early antifungal prophylaxis. It has been mentioned in a study on management of intraabdominal candidiasis (IAC) in clinical settings, that there is urgent need to elaborate the recommendations for IAC management suggested by multidisciplinary expertise panel. It has also been suggested that the restricted use of central venous catheters in hospitals and shortening the stay in ICU may help in reducing the development in invasive candidiasis.

Diabetes

Diabetes is a multisystemic disorder which is characterized by insufficiency of insulin secretion or resistance to the metabolic action of insulin on target tissues. Poor glycemic control in diabetic patients increases susceptibility to candidal infections. The incidence of diabetic population is expected to increase from 171 million in 2000 to 366 million by 2030. The prevalence of candidiasis in diabetic patients is 31.4%. Diabetic patients have increased Candida colonization in oral mucosa in comparison with normal individuals. It has been estimated that diabetic patients have highly glycosylated hemoglobin which can play as important factor for candidal infections and there is a formation of chemically reversible glycosylated products with salivary glucose and proteins in tissues during hyperglycemic episodes. The accumulation of glycosylation products on buccal epithelial cells may result in increasing the number of available receptors for Candida and thus candidiasis. The main factors contributing to oral Candida colonization in case of diabetes mellitus are diabetic type, glycemic control and salivary pH.

The secreted acid proteinase might play a role in the pathogenesis of vulvovaginal candidiasis and improvement in the glucose control may reduce the risk of Candida colonization and potentially symptomatic infection. The prevalence of fungal infections in diabetic patients is also a result of immune dysfunction including low complement factor 4, decreased cytokine response after stimulation in humoral innate immunity and decreased functions (chemotaxis, phagocytosis and killing) of diabetic polymorphonuclear cells and diabetic monocytes/macrophages in cellular innate immunity.

It has been found that antifungal agent fluconazole shows alternation in phospholipase production, modification of buccal epithelial cells and reduction in adhesion of *C. albicans* to human buccal epithelial cells in diabetic patients suffering from oral candidiasis. The use and addition of the iron chelator, deferasirox used in the treatment of zygomycosis in diabetic patients, can be a promising compound but additional agents with new targets of action are also needed.

Burn

Nowadays, *C. albicans* is emerging as a major fungal infection in burn wounds in hospitals, which can result in sepsis as one of the principle causes of death after a severe burn. The incidence of

Candida infections in burn wounds is 35.6%. The burn wound represents a favorable site for fungal infections as they are exposed and serves for opportunistic colonization of fungal infections. The other factors which can favor for infection are age of the patient, extent of injury and depth of the burn wound along with the type, number of microbe attacking the patient, enzyme and toxin production, and motility which determines the likelihood of invasive burn wound infection. The risk factors for invasion are severity of illness, total parenteral nutrition, antibiotics, burns, central venous lines, and immunosuppression. The prevalence of invasive candidiasis in burn cases varies widely and accounts for 3-23% of severe infection with 14 to 70% mortality rate. The detection of fungal infection usually occurs after 14 days of injury. In a study by Kobayashi et al. it has been suggested that burn-associated CD301 type 2 T cells may play a role on the increased susceptibility of burned patients to *C. albicans* infection Nitric oxide nanoparticle has been shown to have antifungal activity and can be used for treatment of cutaneous burn infections and wounds. Nowadays, Serum (1→3)-β-D-glucan (BG) is increasingly used as diagnostic marker for invasive fungal infections.

Neonates and Childhood

Candidal colonization in neonates is a result of vertical transmission from mother infected with candidiasis. The prevalence of candidal infections in neonates is 6.5%. *Candida* colonization which is the first step towards Candida development occurs at rectal sites in neonates. There is an increase in prevalence of fungal arthritis in premature infants with incidence of 10-25%. The other risk factors are long term steroid and antibiotic therapy, immunospression, hyperalimentation, gastrointestinal defects etc. Diaper dermatitis is very common among neonates. which occur due to prolonged exposure to humidity, increased skin pH, feces and urine-induced irritation and zinc deficiency. Thus, secondary infections can be caused by *Candida* when dermatitis remains for more than 3 days. Candidal infections in childhood can be cutaneous, mucosal or systemic candidiasis. Septicaemia in neonatal ICUs occurs due to candidal infections and may affect 1.6-12.9% of very low birth weight infants.

Fluconazole is an effective drug for these infections along with antifungal prophylaxis which includes hygiene regimens, mycological surveillance and application of oral antimycotics.

Pregnancy

This condition can serve as a risk factor for vaginal candidiasis. It has been found that there is more prevalence of *Candida* vaginal colonization in a comparative study on *Candida* infections in pregnant and non-pregnant women. This colonization can result in complications related to delivery. The incidence of *Candida* infections in pregnancy is 27.8%. The most dominant *Candida* is *C. albicans* which has 66.3% prevalence when isolated from Tanzanian pregnant women suffering from vaginal candidiasis. The main cause of prevalence of candidiasis is the disruption of vaginal normal flora. During pregnancy the risk of vaginal thrush increases, possibly due to changes in hormone production, leading to increased glycogen content in the vagina. The effect of vaginal candidiasis in pregnancy is the abnormal vaginal discharge.

The promising treatment of vulvovaginal candidiasis during pregnancy is antifungal testing and determination of virulence factors. It has been suggested that application of gynazol can be recommended in case of recurrent vaginal Candida infection. It has also been reported that *C. albicans* isolated from vaginal exudates in pregnant women is more susceptible to antifungal drugs.

Other Factors

Hydrochloric acid, bile juices and pancreatic enzymes are digestive secretions which play an important role in digesting the food in the gastrointestinal tract of humans. They maintain the integrity of small intestine and prevent the growth of microorganisms such as *Candida* into the absorptive sites in gastrointestinal tracts. But due to intake of antacids, antiulcer drugs and decreased secretion of digestive juices, *Candida* gets opportunity to overgrow in the stomach.

The other factor is the impaired liver function in which the liver is not able to perform its function of detoxification. The accumulated toxins are absorbed by intestine and make the individual more sensitive to chemicals. This stimulates the overgrowth of *Candida* and causes chronic candidiasis in digestive tract. Sucrose, honey, maple syrup, refined sugars, fruit juice, has an important.

Role in functioning as growth enhancers for microbes: Foods with high content of yeast and fungi like cheeses, alcoholic beverages and dried fruits favor the growth of *Candida*. Essential nutrients like magnesium, vitamins A and B6, selenium, zinc, folic acid and essential fatty acids are found to be deficit in chronic candidiasis. The use of drugs and chemical compounds hampers the functioning of liver which results in toxin accumulation thereby altering the bowel micro flora. The balance of micro flora is important in maintaining the nutritional status, cholesterol metabolism, immune system function, carcinogenic agents and aging. The hormonal imbalance, chronic stress also favors the above mentioned conditions which results in overgrowth of *Candida*.

Superficial Mycoses: Dermatophytosis

Fungal skin infections are categorized into superficial and deep, with superficial infections defined as those limited to the stratum corneum of the epidermis, or to the hair and nails. The three most common types of superficial mycoses are dermatophytosis, diseases caused by Malassezia and superficial candidiasis, while the least common are tinea nigra, black and white piedra, and the infections caused by nondermatophytic molds. This chapter will focus on the superficial dermatophytoses.

Superficial fungal infections are some of the most common dermatologic diseases seen worldwide. It is estimated that between 13.8 and 20% of the population has had a dermatophyte infection and approximately 12-13% have onychomycosis.

Dermatophytosis is an infection caused by fungi from three genera, namely Microsporum, Trichophyton, and Epidermophyton. Infections caused by these organisms are referred to as tinea which precedes the Latin name for the site which they involve, i.e. tinea capitis is a dermatophyte infection involving the scalp. The most common system to classify these organisms is based upon mode of transmission; geophilic (found in soil and infect both animals and humans), zoophilic (found on animals, but can be transmitted to humans), and anthropophilic (found on humans). The most common dermatophytes that result in disease in humans are summarized in below Table.

Species	Incidence	Natural habitat	Special features	Associated condition
Epidermophyton floccosum	Common	Humans	Third most common organism	Tinea cruris, pedis, manuum, and onychomycosis
Microsporum audouinii	Less common*	Humans	Ectothrix, Wood lamp green fluorescence	Tinea capitis—more common in Europe
Microsporum canis	Common	Cats	Ectothrix, Wood lamp green fluorescence, associated with pet exposure	Tinea capitis—second most common. 10% can result in kerionTinea barbae
Microsporum ferrugineum	Common	Humans		Tinea capitis
Microsporum gypseum	Common	Soil	Outdoor or occupational exposure	Inflammatory lesions
Trichophyton rubrum	Very common	Humans	Most common organism worldwide, 58%	Tinea corporis, cruris, pedis, manuum, and onychomycosis and Majocchi granuloma
Trichophyton tonsurans	Common	Humans	Endothrix, 3%	Tinea capitis—majority of cases in United States. Common cause of tinea corporis worldwide
Trichophyton violaceum	Less common	Humans	Endothrix	Tinea capitis—endothrix
Trichophyton mentagrophytes var interdigitale	Common	Humans	Second most common organism causing tinea corporis and pedis, 27%	Tinea corporis, cruris, pedis (interdigital), manuum, and onychomycosis
Trichophyton mentagrophytes var mentagrophytes	Common	Mice, rodents		Inflammatory tinea pedis and barbae, dermatophytid reaction
Trichophyton verrucosum	Common	Cattle	7%	Tinea barbae, capitis, and kerion
Trichophyton nanum	Less common	Pigs		Tinea capitis, corporis, and cruris
Trichophyton simii	Less common*	Monkeys	Asia	Tinea capitis
Trichophyton equinum	Less common	Horse		Tinea corporis
Trichophyton concentricum	Rare*	Humans	Genetic and immunologic susceptibility, geographic restriction	Tinea imbricata
Trichophyton schoenleinii	Rare*	Humans	Endothrix, blue-white fluorescence with Wood lamp	Favus
Trichophyton soudanense	Rare*	Humans	Africa	Tinea capitis

*Geographically restricted.

Mucosal and Cutaneous Infections

Cutaneous fungal infections, also known as mycoses, are common and superficial infections caused by fungi invading the skin and its appendages, which include the hair, scalp, and nails.

Now, let's review some physiology. Normally, the skin surface is colonized by a huge number of microorganisms that make up the normal skin flora. This flora has a healthy balance that consists mostly of bacteria, such as Staphylococcus epidermidis, as well as low amounts of certain fungi, such as *Candida albicans*, Malassezia, and dermatophytes like Trichophyton. These microorganisms are typically non-pathogenic, meaning that they don't cause any disease. In fact, they are beneficial, since they serve as a physical and competitive barrier that helps prevent pathogenic microorganisms from invading and infecting the skin.

Okay, so cutaneous fungal infections are typically caused by a disruption of the healthy balance of the skin flora. Now, clients can develop different infections based on the causative fungus. The most common ones include candidiasis, which is caused by an overgrowth of *Candida albicans*; as well as tinea or pityriasis versicolor, which is caused by Malassezia furfur; and tinea infections, which are caused by a variety of dermatophyte fungi.

Risk factors of fungal infections include medications like antibiotics or glucocorticoids, poor personal hygiene, as well as warm and humid environments, in addition to close contact with animals, such as dogs, cats, cows, and goats. Additional risk factors include obesity, diabetes mellitus, and being immunocompromised; as well as high estrogen levels due to oral contraceptive use, estrogen therapy, or pregnancy.

So, cutaneous fungal infections occur when the healthy balance of the skin flora gets disrupted, which may allow the fungi in the skin to overgrow. In most cases, a healthy immune system is able to notice and stop this, keeping the fungi under control. However, in some cases, fungi manage to persist, and ultimately cause an infection. Typically, cutaneous fungal infections are superficial and localized; but in certain cases, such as in clients who are severely immunocompromised, fungi may also cause more serious invasive infections, spreading to the bloodstream or to other tissues and organs.

Now, the clinical manifestations of cutaneous fungal infections may vary according to the causative fungus. Candidiasis typically presents as a well-defined erythematous area that's often itchy, most often involving moist intertriginous areas where two skin surfaces rub together, such as the axillae and groin folds. In babies and young children who wear diapers, Candida infection may cause diaper dermatitis, which presents as a sharp red patch with surrounding or satellite eruptions.

On the other hand, tinea or pityriasis versicolor causes patches of hypo- or hyperpigmentation of the skin, most often involving the neck, chest, back, and arms.

Lastly, tinea infections usually present as an erythematous scaly plaque with a characteristic ring-like appearance; these lesions are sometimes itchy. Now, depending on the body site affected, tinea infections can be classified as tinea capitis when it involves the scalp; tinea barbae when it involves the beard and mustache area, also called barber's itch; tinea cruris when it involves the groin area, also called jock itch; tinea pedis when it involves the toes or feet, also called athlete's foot; tinea unguium when it involves the toenails or fingernails, also known as onychomycosis; and finally, tinea corporis when the infection affects any site of the body, excluding the scalp, face or beard, groin, and hands, feet, or nails.

The mucosal surfaces of the body are colonised by a diverse microbiota. Tremendous advances have been made in our understanding of the microbes that colonise mucosal surfaces and while the predominant numbers of colonising microbial species are bacterial in origin, the role of fungi in these polymicrobial communities is significant.

Approximately 20 species of *Candida* fungi are known to be pathogenic to humans. Localised overgrowth of *Candida* fungi on mucosal surfaces results in the development of candidiasis at disparate mucosal sites in the body (oral, gastrointestinal, vaginal), causing morbidity in otherwise healthy individuals, and deep-seated invasive infections that threaten mortality in the absence of effective immune defence. The direct and indirect mechanisms used by *Candida* species to colonise, damage, and breach mucosal barriers are discussed by Richardson et al. together with a review of secreted virulence factors and their contribution to mucosal interactions. This includes recent findings relevant to the activity of candidalysin, the first fungal peptide toxin identified in any human fungal pathogen. The host immune response to invasive fungi is a critical determinant of clearance from the body. Recent years have seen significant advances in our understanding of innate mucosal immunity to *C. albicans*. In their review, Verma et al. explore the innate mechanisms of epithelial defence against Candida fungi with an emphasis on responses to *C. albicans*. The authors evaluate the role of soluble host factors (cytokines, chemokines, antimicrobial peptides, and alarmins) in effective defence and highlight the role of innate immunity mediated by haematopoietic cells.

Aspergillus fumigatus is a common airborne saprophytic fungus. During its life cycle, *A. fumigatus* releases conidia into the atmosphere that are subsequently inhaled into the lungs where they cause a complex range of debilitating respiratory infections in patients with compromised immunity. In their review, Bertuzzi et al. explore the temporal and mechanistic events that underpin attachment and uptake of *A. fumigatus* by the respiratory epithelium, the contribution of these processes to respiratory aspergilloses, and epithelial responses to the fungus. Differential cellular responses to *A. fumigatus* morphotypes are discussed by the authors as well as current opinions regarding the role of epithelial uptake as a curative or pathogenic process. The adaptive T-Helper (Th) immune responses to *A. fumigatus* are explored in detail by Dewi et al, who review the factors that influence effective adaptive clearance (Th1/Th17) and allergic hypersensitivity/detrimental immune pathology (Th2/Th17). The authors also discuss the role of regulatory T-cells in this context and explore the challenges associated with the development of effective immunotherapy.

The basidiomycete *Cryptococcus neoformans* causes disease in otherwise healthy individuals and those with compromised immunity. As the onset of cryptococcosis is typically associated with HIV positive individuals and hence defective adaptive immunity, mucosal defence against *C. neoformans* is somewhat understudied by comparison. Taylor-Smith reviews the interactions that occur between *C. neoformans* and epithelial cells that lead to fungal adherence and internalisation into the respiratory mucosa. The importance of bronchial and alveolar epithelial responses in driving innate defence against infecting fungus is explored together with a discussion of fungal responses in the respiratory niche. The recent advances in adaptive immunity to *C. neoformans* are considered by Mukaremera and Nielsen, who discuss the complex and varied cellular and antibody responses to the fungus. The authors also evaluate the role of protective cytokines, and present current models that describe adaptive immune responses *to C. neoformans* in mice and humans.

Fungi of the order Mucorales (predominantly *Rhizopus*, *Mucor*, and *Lichtheimia* species) are the cause of mucormycosis, an aggressive, devastating invasive fungal disease with a mortality rate of 50–100%. The innate and adaptive immune defence mechanisms that are brought to bear against Mucorales are discussed by Ghuman and Voelz, who describe the role of immune cells and platelets in antifungal defence together with the challenges faced when clearing Mucorales from the body, a process whose efficacy is influenced by the developmental stage of Mucorales sporangiospores.

Systemic Mycoses

Primary Pathogens and Opportunistic Pathogens

Systemic mycoses are fungal infections affecting internal organs. In the right circumstances the fungi enter the body via the lungs, through the gut, paranasal sinuses or skin. The fungi can then spread via the bloodstream to multiple organs including the skin, often causing multiple organs to fail and eventually resulting in the death of the patient.

Causes of Systemic Mycoses

Patients who are immunocompromised are more predisposed to systemic mycoses, but they can develop in otherwise healthy patients. Systemic mycoses can be split between two main varieties, endemic respiratory infections and opportunistic infections.

Endemic Respiratory Infections

Fungi that can cause systemic infection in people with normal immune function as well as those who are immune-compromised include:

- Histoplasma capsulatum (causing histoplasmosis),
- Coccidioides immitis (causing coccidioidomycosis),
- Blastomyces dermatitidis (causing blastomycosis),
- Paracoccidioides brasiliensis (causing paracoccidioidomycosis) and
- Talaromyces marneffei (causing talaromycosis).

These fungi are found in soil and wood debris. Histoplasma is prevalent in Southern USA, Central America, South America, Africa and Asia. Coccidioides and Paracoccidioides are prevalent in Southern USA and Central America. Blastomyces is most often found in North America. *Talaromyces marneffei* (formerly known as *Penicillium marneffei*) is endemic in tropical Southeast Asia.

Opportunistic Infections

Fungi that only result in systemic infection in immunocompromised or sick people include:

- Candida species including non-albicans candida (causing candidiasis).
- Aspergillus species (causing aspergillosis).
- Cryptococcus (causing cryptococcosis).
- Zygomycetes (causing zygomycosis).

These fungi are found in or on normal skin, decaying vegetable matter, and bird droppings respectively, but not exclusively. They are present throughout the world.

Susceptible to Systemic Mycoses

Immune compromised people are at risk of systemic mycoses. Immunodeficiency can result from:

- Human immunodeficiency virus (HIV) infection.
- Systemic malignancy (cancer).
- Neutropenia (low white blood cell count).
- Organ transplant recipients and following haematological stem cell transplant.
- After a major surgical operation.
- Poorly controlled diabetes mellitus.
- Adult-onset immunodeficiency syndrome.
- Very old or very young.

Clinical Features of Systemic Mycoses

The clinical features of a systemic mycosis depend on the specific infection and which organs have been affected. Infections in people with normal immune function may result in very minor symptoms or none at all (this is called subclinical infection). General symptoms of illness may include:

- Fever.
- Cough.
- Loss of appetite.

Lungs

Invasive lung mycoses typically result in a progressive dry cough, shortness of breath, pain when taking a deep breath and fever. These symptoms may progress to the point of life-threatening acute respiratory distress syndrome. Haemoptysis (the coughing up of blood) is also sometimes seen, particularly if any inflammation of the large airways is present.

Bone

Bone infection can develop from spread through the blood or rarely via direct spread from an overlying ulcer and infected skin. Fever and pain in the affected bone are cardinal symptoms. This would usually be investigated with x-rays, computed tomography (CT) scanning and an aspiration via a needle to obtain a specimen for culture.

Brain

Brain involvement by systemic mycoses has a particularly high mortality. Symptoms suggesting the involvement of the brain include headaches, seizures and deficits in normal brain control over movement or sensation. These are assessed by CT or magnetic resonance imaging (MRI) brain scans and if suggestive, then may be followed up by biopsy of the brain.

Meningitis

Inflammation of the tissue surrounding the brain can develop, particularly with candidiasis and cryptococcosis. Symptoms usually include headache, stiff neck and irritability.

Eyes

Almost any of the eye structures may be infected by mycoses. *Candida spp.* and *Cryptococcus spp.* are the most commonly infecting mycoses. The symptoms depend on which part of the eye is infected but may include visual blurring, dark or black images floating in the visual field, pain and a red eye.

Skin

A variety of skin changes may be seen in association with systemic mycoses. The skin lesions depend partly on which fungus is the cause.

Infection	Clinical features
Candidiasis	• Single or widespread lesions • Small red papules or larger nodules • Purpuric lesions can resemble ecthyma gangrenosum or purpura fulminans
Aspergillosis	• Few or many lesions • May result in rapidly spreading red patch with a necrotic centre (blackened dead tissue) • May resemble pyoderma gangrenosum
Cryptococcosis	• Most often a skin rash is the first sign of infection • Extremely varied appearance • Papules, abscesses, plaques, blisters, sinuses, ulcers, cellulitis or purpura (bleeding into the skin)
Blastomycosis	• Papules, nodules, warty lesions • Pustules, abscesses, ulcers and scars • May cause oral lesions

Histoplasmosis	• Scaly (psoriasis-like) or soft papules, nodules, abscesses, sinuses or ulcers • May cause mouth ulcers • May cause erythema multiforme, erythema nodosum or toxic erythema
Coccidioidomycosis	• Papular lesions, plaques, abscesses, sinuses, ulceration or toxic erythema (a generalized red rash) • Hypersensitivity reactions may result in erythema multiforme
Talaromycosis	• Umbilicated papules and ulcers
Zycomycosis	• Mucorales infection causes plaques, pustules, abscesses and ulcers • Entomophthorales infection causes slowly progressive subcutaneous firm or hard nodules, often affecting the nose or sinuses

Aspergillus Skin Lesion

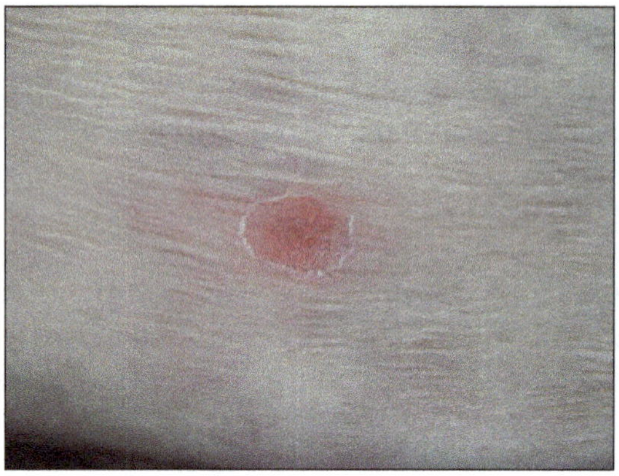

Aspergillus skin lesion.

Tests to Diagnose Systemic Mycoses

The most reliable tests to confirm infection are skin biopsy for histological (microscopic) analysis and fungal culture. Blood can also be cultured.

Treatment for Systemic Mycoses

Once a diagnosis of systemic mycoses has been established the immune compromise should be reversed if possible, for example by discontinuing immune-suppressing medications or at least reducing their dose.

Systemic antifungal medications can also be given. Suitable drugs include:

- Amphotericin B,
- Fluconazole,
- Itraconazole,
- Voriconazole and
- Caspofungin.

The prognosis depends on the patient's immune function and the extent of infection when treatment is started. Despite treatment, many patients die of their infection.

Subcutaneous Mycoses

Subcutaneous mycoses include a heterogeneous group of fungal infections that develop at the site of transcutaneous trauma. The main subcutaneous fungal infections include sporotrichosis, chromoblastomycosis, mycetoma, lobomycosis, phaeohyphomycosis, subcutaneous zygomycosis and Chromoblastomycosis (Verrucous dermatitis).

Aetiological agents include various dematiaceous hyphomycetes associated with soil, especially Phialophora verrucosa.

Clinical Manifestations

Lesions of chromoblastomycosis are most often found on exposed parts of the body and usually start a small scaly papules or nodules which are painless but may be itchy. lesions may gradually arise and as the disease develops rash-like areas enlarge and become raised irregular plaques that are often scaly or verrucose. In long standing infections, lesions may become tumorous and even cauliflower-like in appearance. Other prominent features include epithelial hyperplasia, fibrosis and microabscess formation in the epidermis.

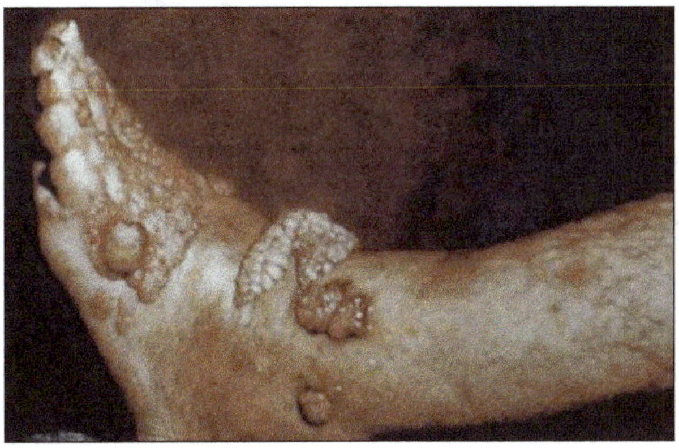

Chromoblastomycosis presenting on the toes, foot.

Laboratory Diagnosis

- Clinical Material: Skin scrapings and/or biopsy.
- Direct Microscopy: (a) Skin scrapings should be examined using 10% KOH and Parker ink or calcofluor white mounts; (b) Tissue sections should be stained using H&E, PAS digest, and Grocott's methenamine silver (GMS).

Skin scrapings from a patient with chromoblastomycosis mounted in 10% KOH and Parker ink solution showing characteristic brown pigmented, planate-dividing, rounde sclerotic bodies (Medlar bodies).

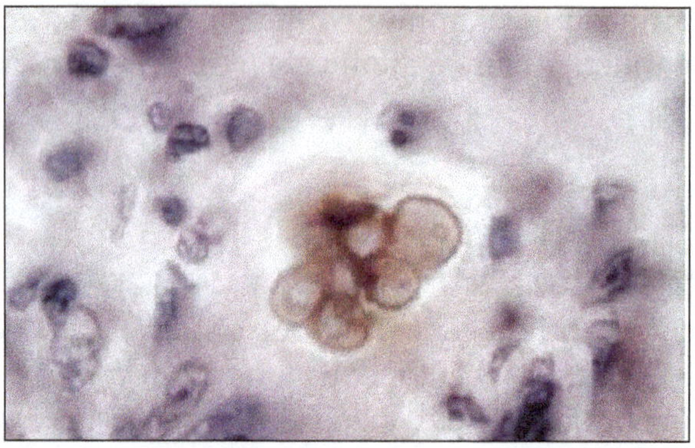

Chromoblastomycosis: Histological sample stained with hematoxylin and eosin showing the brown-pigmented Medlar bodies.

- Culture: Clinical specimens should be inoculated onto primary isolation media, like Sabouraud's dextrose agar.

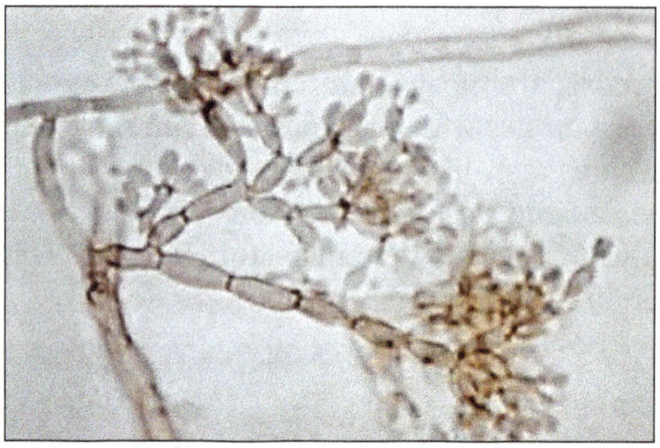

Chromoblastomycosis: Culture stained with 10% KOH revealing the Medlar bodies, muriform bodies or sclerotic cells with round, brown, thick-walled and multi-septate cells.

- Serology: There are currently no commercially available serological procedures for the diagnosis of chromoblastomycosis.

Management

The treatment of chromoblastomycosis has been exceedingly difficult. Successful surgical excision requires the removal of a margin of uninfected tissue to prevent local dissemination. both itraconazole [400 mg/day] and terbinafine [500 mg/ day] for 6 to 12 months have been used successfully for the treatment of chromoblastomycosis.

Lobomycosis (Lacaziosis)

Aetiological agents include Lacazia loboi, the disease has been found in humans and dolphins.

Clinical Manifestations

The initial infection is thought to be caused by traumatic implantation such as an arthropod sting, snake bite, or wound acquired while cutting vegetation. The lesions begin as small, hard nodules and may spread slowly in the dermis and continue to develop over a period of many years. Older lesions become verrucoid and may ulcerate. The disease may be transferred to other areas of the skin by further trauma or autoinoculation. Lesions are usually found on the arms, legs, face or ears.

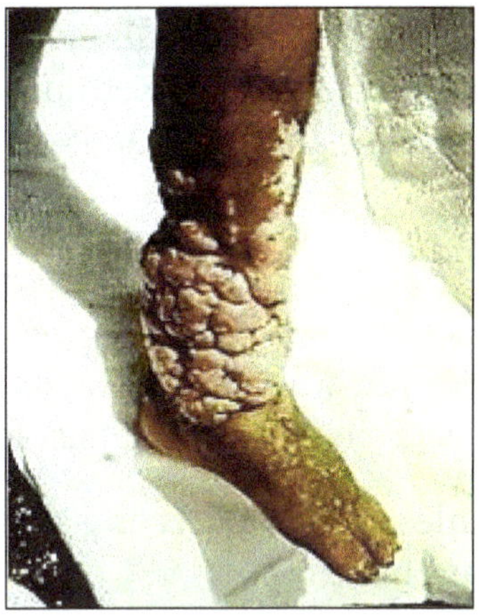

Lobomycosis showing extensive verrucoid lesions on the legs.

The lesions affect mainly exposed areas such as upper and lower limbs and are typically presented as keloid-like lesions

Laboratory Diagnosis

- Clinical material: Tissue sample obtained by curettage or surgical biopsy.
- Direct Microscopy: (a) Tissue can be macerated and mounted in 10% KOH and Parker ink or calcofluor white mounts or (b) Tissue sections should be stained using PAS digest, Grocott's methenamine silver (GMS) or Gram stains.

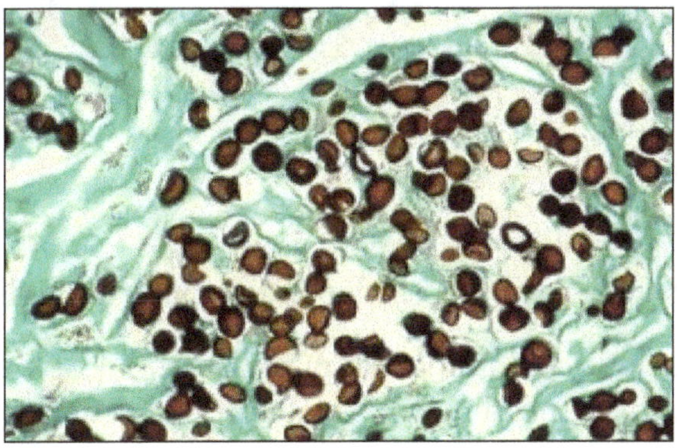

GMS stained tissue specimen showing numerous darkly pigmented yeast-like cells, often in chains, 9-1 μm in size.

- Culture: The aetiologic agent known as "Loboa loboi" remains to be cultured.
- Serology: There are currently no serological tests available

Management

The most successful treatment is for wide surgical excision of the affected area, however care must be taken to prevent contamination of surgical wounds, as relapse is common. Clofazimine at 100-200 mg/day has been used with varying results.

Mycetoma (Maduromycosis)

A mycotic infection of humans and animals Mycetoma are caused by 2 totally different groups of organisms: the first are moulds, and the second are filamentous bacteria in the order Actinomycetales. In the first case they are referred to as eumycetomas, in the second as actinomycetomas characterized by draining sinuses, granules and tumefaction. Aetiological agents include Madurella, Fusarium, Aspergillus etc.

Clinical Manifestations

Mycetoma is more common in men than women, particularly those aged 20 to 50. It generally presents as a single lesion on an exposed site and may persist for years. Two thirds arise on the foot.

- It starts as a small hard painless lump under the skin. It grows slowly but eventually involves underlying muscles and bones.
- The middle of the lesion caves in ulcerates and discharges pus, which contains grains.
- Granules which vary in size, colour and degree of hardness, depending on the aetiologic species. These grains are the hallmark of mycetoma.

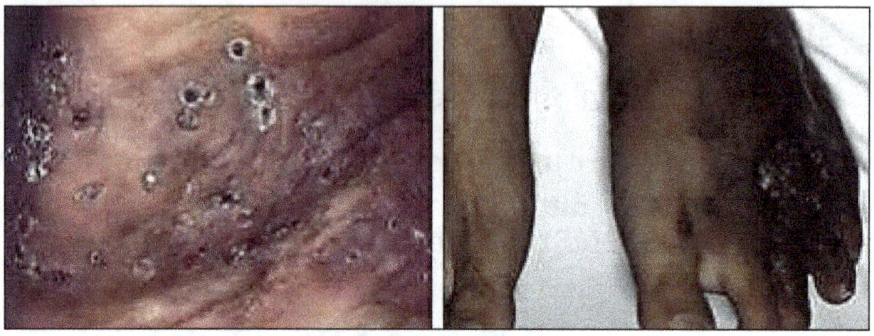

Sinuses from Nocardia.

Laboratory Diagnosis

- Clinical Material: Tissue biopsy or excised sinus, fluid containing the granules which vary in size, colour and degree of hardness, depending on the aetiologic species.
- Direct Microscopy: fluid containing the granules should be examined using either 10% KOH and Parker ink or calcofluor white mounts, and tissue sections should be stained using H&E, PAS digest, and Grocott' smethenamine silver (GMS). The colour of the grains may suggest the likely diagnosis; black grains suggest a fungal infection,

Microscopy using potassium hydroxide (KOH) confirms the diagnosis and type of mycetoma.

- Actinomycotic grains contain very fine filaments.
- Fungal grains contain short hyphae (branched filaments) that are often swollen
- Culture: Clinical specimens should be inoculated onto primary isolation media, like Sabouraud's dextrose agar. Several agar plates are cultured at 25-30 degrees celcius and 37 degrees celcius for up to six weeks. Fungi grow more quickly than actinomycetes.

- Serology: There are currently no commercially available serological procedures for the diagnosis of mycetoma.

Treatment of Mycetoma

Actinomycetoma

- Streptomycin injections
- Amikacin, rifampicin and tetracycline.

Eumycetoma is more difficult to treat.

- Itraconazole and ketoconazole
- Surgery to remove the affected tissue completely. These may mean amputation if bone is involved

Emerging Fungal Infections

The epidemiology of invasive fungal infection is evolving. Yeasts other than *Candida albicans* and molds other than *Aspergillus fumigatus* have emerged as significant causes of invasive mycoses in severely immunocompromised patients. Although, in some instances, these changes may be related to medical interventions, such as the use of antifungal agents in prophylaxis, in the majority of cases, they seem to be a consequence of changes in the host, such as more-severe immunosuppression or different types of immunosuppression impacting both risk periods and the infections that occur. These factors have altered the epidemiology of infection in organ transplant recipients, premature newborns, and critically ill patients. This review discusses the epidemiology of some fungal infections that have emerged in the past few years, with an emphasis on the potential factors associated with their emergence and on practical implications of these epidemiological changes.

The epidemiology of invasive fungal infection has changed during the past 20 years. The incidence has increased, and the population of patients at risk has expanded to include those with a broad list of medical conditions, such as solid-organ and hematopoietic stem cell transplantation (HSCT), cancer, receipt of immunosuppressive therapy, AIDS, premature birth, advanced age, and major surgery. Furthermore, the etiology of these infections has changed. In the 1980s, yeasts (particularly *Candida albicans*) were the most common causative agents of invasive mycoses. In recent years, molds have become more frequent in certain groups of patients, such as HSCT recipients, and, in patients in whom candidiasis is still the most frequent invasive mycosis, non-*albicans* species of *Candida* account for >50% of infections. In addition, infections caused by other yeasts, such as *Trichosporon* species, have been reported. Among molds, reports of aspergillosis caused by non-fumigatus species of *Aspergillus*, *zygomycosis*, and infection caused by hyaline and black molds have been increasing in number. The exact reasons for these changes are not completely clear. In some circumstances, they may be related to specific medical interventions, such as antifungal prophylaxis and the use of medical devices. However, in the majority of the cases, they seem to be a consequence of changes in the host, such as more-severe immunosuppression or different types of immunosuppression impacting both risk periods and the infections that occur.

The term "emerging infection" may be used to denote an infection that has newly appeared in the population or one that is rapidly increasing in incidence or geographic range. Now we will discuss the epidemiology of some fungal infections that have emerged in the past few years, with an emphasis on the potential factors associated with their emergence and on practical implications of these epidemiological changes. A summary of the suggested therapy for these infections is shown in table.

Table: Treatments of choice for emerging fungal infections.

Causative agent, by type	Treatment
Yeasts	
Candida glabrata	Caspofungin
Candida rugosa	Fluconazole, amphotericin Ba
Trichosporon species	Fluconazole
Cryptococcus gattii	Amphotericin B, fluconazole
Molds	
Aspergillus terreus	Voriconazole
Zygomycetes	Amphotericin B at high doses, lipid amphotericin B, posaconazole
Fusarium species	Lipid amphotericin B, Voriconazole
Scedosporium apiospermum	Voriconazole, itraconazole
Scedosporium prolificans	Voriconazole

Emerging Yeasts: Fungemia

As mentioned above, *C. albicans* has been regarded as the most common agent of invasive yeast infection. With the introduction and widespread use of fluconazole, the overall incidence of candidemia has decreased, with a reduction of infections caused by *C. albicans* and an increase of infections caused by *Candida glabrata*. *C. glabrata* has emerged as the secondmost common agent of candidemia in the United States since the early 1990s. In addition, *C. glabrata* has been recently associated with oropharyngeal candidiasis in patients receiving radiotherapy for head and neck cancer. A major problem with infection due to *C. glabrata* is its decreased susceptibility to fluconazole. With the newer azoles, cross-resistance is also a concern, because the main mechanism of resistance to fluconazole is the over-expression of multidrug efflux pumps. In a large study that evaluated 610 isolates of *C. glabrata* obtained from patients from different parts of the world with invasive infections, the percentages of strains susceptible to posaconazole, ravuconazole, and voriconazole (with MICs of <1μg/mL) were 85.4%, 90.7%, and 92.8%, respectively. More importantly, among 46 fluconazole-resistant isolates of C. glabrata, only 13% were susceptible to voriconazole, 4% were susceptible to posaconazole, and 8.7% were susceptible to ravuconazole. The potential for the emergence of voriconazole-resistant *C. glabrata* as a threat to people receiving voriconazole therapy is an issue that has been raised in a case study of breakthrough infections at a single health care center.

In some parts of the world, especially in Latin American countries, *Candida parapsilosis* and *Candida tropicalis* preempt *C. glabrata* as the second leading cause of candidemia. Although reasons for the emergence of these organisms are not known, risk factors such as the use of intravenous catheters, contamination of infusate, and colonization of health care workers have been implicated in *C. parapsilosis* infection, instead of drug-induced selection pressure. Geographical differences outline the complexity of epidemiology; multiple factors, including the specialties of regional medical centers, patterns of practice, and host factors, likely support the emergence of different Candida species as predominant pathogens. Data from preliminary results of in vitro susceptibility testing with the echinocandins suggest that some isolates of *C. parapsilosis* exhibit higher MICs than do other *Candida* species. Although the clinical consequences of these findings are not known, the recent report of the development of multiple-echinocandin resistance during exposure to these agents is a concern, especially because these agents have been increasingly used as primary therapy for candidemia.

Candida rugosa has been rarely reported as a human pathogen. In 1994, an outbreak of fungemia due to this organism was reported in a burn unit in the United States. No obvious source was identified, and the authors associated its occurrence with the use of topical nystatin in burn wounds. More recently, another outbreak was reported in an intensive care unit of a tertiary care hospital in Brazil during a surveillance study of candidemia in 6 institutions from 3 different cities. Six cases were identified within a 4-month period. All patients had coexisting exposures that were very usual for patients with candidemia, such as the presence of a central venous catheter, antibiotic therapy, surgery, and mechanical ventilation. Again, no source of the infections was identified, but DNA typing showed that all isolates were genotypically related. In a subsequent study performed in the same unit, 349 patients were prospectively evaluated with biweekly cultures of samples from sites of colonization to investigate the predictive value of *Candida* colonization in the diagnosis of candidemia. Surprisingly, 15% of the 1400 cultures with positive results grew *C. rugosa*, which accounted for 43.7% of the 32 episodes of candidemia (data not shown). Therefore, although most reports of infection due to *C. rugosa* occurred in the context of outbreaks, there are data suggesting that this species may be endemic to some institutions.

Trichosporon species have been associated with fungemia and disseminated infection since the late 1980s. This organism most frequently causes disseminated infection in neutropenic patients with cancer. By contrast, in a recent report from a single cancer center, most infections were catheter-related fungemias. The reasons for these changes are not clear, but it is possible that the widespread use of fluconazole may have played some role, because this agent is active in vitro against Trichosporon species. More recently, trichosporonosis has been reported in neonates. Most patients were born prematurely, with a mean birth-weight <1000 g. The majority of cases were of disseminated infection, and, in >90% of cases, the fungus was isolated from the respiratory tract.

Other Emerging Yeasts

Cryptococcal infections occur with a near worldwide distribution in immunosuppressed hosts. Infections typically are caused by *Cryptococcus neoformans*; however, *Cryptococcus gattii* causes disease in immunocompetent people in a geographically restricted fashion, with most cases occurring in Australia. A notable recent development is the recognition of *C. gattii* as a cause of invasive infection in animals and immunocompetent people on Vancouver Island, Western Canada. An outbreak that now involves >100 people has been occurring since 1999 (K. Bartlett, personal communication). The organism, which is thought to thrive only in tropical regions, was recovered in the environment in a temperate climatic zone. Precisely why the organism emerged in this region has not been determined; it has been postulated that environmental factors—namely, a regional warming trend—may support its environmental propagation. More studies are warranted to determine the clinical significance of this fungus and to define how the environmental factors may play a role in supporting the emergence of pathogenic fungi.

Emerging Molds

The epidemiology of mold infections has changed substantially in the past 10 years. The incidence of invasive aspergillosis (IA) has increased significantly , and infections caused by molds that exhibit resistance to conventional antifungal agents, such as *Fusarium* species and the Zygomycetes, have been increasingly reported.

Most cases of IA occur in patients with hematologic malignancies or in transplant recipients (especially recipients of HSCTs, lung transplants, and liver transplants). In the former group, acute myeloid leukemia is the most frequent underlying condition, but, in recent years, IA has been increasingly diagnosed in patients with multiple myeloma. In a study of recipients of HSCTs, the risk of IA was 4.5 times greater in patients with multiple myeloma, compared with the risk for patients with chronic myeloid leukemia in the chronic phase. In an epidemiologic study of 15 health care centers, 31 cases of IA in patients with multiple myeloma were identified in a 12-year period. Of these cases, 74% were diagnosed in the last 5 years of the study. Remarkably, neutropenia was present in only 51% of patients with IA and myeloma, and all nonneutropenic patients had received high doses of corticosteroids. In a study of 69 autopsies performed on patients with multiple myeloma, IA had been diagnosed in 53% of the 38 deaths associated with infection, and IA was identified by autopsy in 45% of recipients of allogeneic HSCT, 21% of recipients of autologous HSCT, and 25% of patients who had completed a course of chemotherapy. The increased number of reports of IA in patients with multiple myeloma may be related to changes in its treatment, with the incorporation of the concept of sequential aggressive therapy into the practice of intensive chemotherapy, double autologous transplantation, and nonmyeloablative allogeneic transplantation.

The time of onset of IA in recipients of allogeneic stem-cell engraftment has changed. Now, the infection typically occurs late, after HSCT is complete, when recipients are receiving immunosuppressive drugs (especially high doses of corticosteroids) for the treatment of graft-versus-host disease. This shift is likely caused by changes in transplant procedures that have resulted in a reduction in the duration of neutropenia and an increase in the incidence and severity of graft-versushost disease. Examples of changes in transplantation procedures include the use of peripheral blood instead of bone marrow as the source of stem cells, transplantation with reduced-intensity conditioning regimens (e.g., nonmyeloablative transplant), mismatched and unrelated transplant donors, donor lymphocyte infusion, and the use of monoclonal antibodies, such as infliximab and alemtuzumab.

Late onset of IA has also been reported to have occurred in liver transplant recipients for a number of reasons, including a better survival of the organism in the early posttransplantation period, late occurrence of cytomegalovirus disease, and a higher number of patients with late allograft dysfunction.

Another trend of IA is the increasing number of reports of infections caused by species other than *Aspergillus fumigatus*. Of particular concern is *Aspergillus terreus*, because of its in vitro resistance and poor clinical response to amphotericin B. In a single-center study, *A. terreus* accounted for 2.1% of cases of IA in 1996 and 10.2% of cases in 2001. The reasons why the relative incidence of infection due to *A. terreus* is increasing are not clear. The prognosis of IA caused by *A. terreus* is poor, with an overall mortality rate of 66%, and patients treated with voriconazole seem to have a better outcome. Finally, infections caused by a recently recognized species of *Aspergillus* have been reported. The organism, which, according to classical morphological typing methods, is typically identified as *A. fumigatus*, clusters as a unique species with multilocus sequence typing, supporting the proposed designation of "*Aspergillus lentulus*." Representative isolates have now been identified in multiple US health care centers and in Australia; the organism may be of particular interest because isolates exhibit low susceptibility to multiple antifungals in vitro. The clinical significance of this organism is a topic of current study.

Zygomycosis has emerged as a significant infection in transplant recipients. In a multicenter survey of fungal infections in transplant recipients, the proportion of cases of zygomycosis increased from 4% to 25% between 2001 and 2003. Among HSCT recipients, there were 4 cases of zygomycosis among recipients of 4358 transplants (0.09% of recipients) between March 2001 and April 2002, compared with 11 cases in recipients of 6660 transplants (0.17% of recipients) between May 2002 and June 2003. Multivariate analysis of risk factors associated with zygomycosis, compared with those associated with IA, revealed that the previous exposure to voriconazole was significant for both HSCT (OR, 7.7) and solid-organ transplantation (OR, 10.7). The association between the use of voriconazole and zygomycosis is further supported by 4 reports of cases of breakthrough zygomycosis in 15 patients receiving voriconazole therapy, as well as a single-center case-control study that identified the previous exposure to voriconazole as a significant risk factor for zygomycosis by multivariate analysis. Although the use of voriconazole may have contributed to the occurrence of zygomycosis, other factors may be equally important. As pointed out by Kauffman, there are some data indicating that the incidence of zygomycosis was increasing before the introduction of voriconazole in clinical practice. Other factors likely associated with the recent increase include the severity and type of immunosuppression. In one recent report, all patients who developed zygomycosis after neutrophil engraftment had severe graft-versus-host disease and had previously received high doses of corticosteroids and/or antithyomocyte globulin. Another explanation for the increase in the incidence of zygomycosis is the potential decrease in IA-related mortality in most recent years. It is possible that the control of a highly aggressive infection has allowed patients to live long enough to develop a subsequent infection with persistent immunosuppression. With this in mind, zygomycosis may be considered the "third threat" for fungal infections in recipients of allogeneic HSCTs, after infections caused by *C. albicans* and *A. fumigatus*, each of which are more likely to occur in patients who are not receiving an effective preventative regimen.

There have been an increasing number of reports of fusariosis in immunocompromised patients. Data from a multicenter retrospective study of fusariosis in HSCT recipients showed that the rate of infection has increased over time. The main reason for this increase seems to be severe immunosuppression, because the incidence of fusariosis was higher in transplant recipients with mismatched donors and because most patients had either severe neutropenia or graft-versus-host disease. Indeed, a significant number of cases were diagnosed very late after transplantation (>1 year) and none of these patients was neutropenic. This population of patients could be at risk for fusariosis because of severe T cell–mediated immunodeficiency.

In addition to these infections, a broad list of other fungi, including *Scedosporium* species, *Acremonium* species, and *Phialemonium* species, has been occasionally reported as causes of infection in immunocompromised patients. An increase in the incidence of non-*Aspergillus* mold infections has been observed in recipients of liver transplants and HSCTs. This increase in incidence is likely a reflection of more severe immunosuppression.

Fungal Mycotoxins

Mycotoxins are chemicals produced by fungi (molds) under certain conditions. They are not essential for fungal growth or reproduction, and are toxic to animals or humans. Scientists do not yet know how many mycotoxins may exist, even though more than 250 have been detected. They represent many different kinds of chemicals. For many, if not most, their toxicological characteristics have not been fully determined.

Diseases in animals caused by mycotoxins are called mycotoxicoses. There are many different kinds of mycotoxicoses because there are many different kinds of mycotoxins.

It is not intended to allow animal owners to diagnose cases of mycotoxicoses without consulting a veterinarian. Diagnosing mycotoxicoses is not easy. Other diseases besides mycotoxicoses can cause similar clinical signs or lesions, and the expertise of a veterinarian is vital to accurate diagnoses. Otherwise, valuable resources may be worthlessly expended treating wrong diseases.

The medical vocabulary used here may not be familiar to some. Definitions of unfamiliar words may be found in medical dictionaries.

Mycotoxicoses and Mycoses

Diseases called mycotoxicoses and mycoses are sometimes confused. They are not the same. Diseases caused by mycotoxins are called mycotoxicoses. Diseases caused by mold infections are called mycoses.

Mycotoxicoses occur when mycotoxins enter the body, usually by consumption of contaminated feed. Ill health is caused by actions of mycotoxins on cells in the body. Mycotoxicoses are not contagious, nor is there significant stimulation of the immune system.

Mycoses occur when molds infect tissues of the body. They can be contagious. Molds begin to grow in or on the body after the infections are established. There may be stimulation of the immune system. Common mycoses include athlete's foot and ringworm.

Diagnosis and Treatment of Mycotoxicoses

Different mycotoxins cause different diseases. Although they all are called mycotoxicoses, they are very different from each other.

Modern agricultural practices make acute mycotoxicoses with high death loss (mortality) rare. Chronic mycotoxicoses are often suspected when clinical signs include poor performance, ill thrift, or increased incidence of infectious diseases. Establishing cause and effect relationships between consumption of mycotoxin-contaminated feed and vague chronic conditions is very difficult.

Diagnosis of mycotoxicoses is usually not very easy. Exposure cannot be established by detection of mycotoxins in tissues from animals suspected of being poisoned by mycotoxins because analytical services for detection of mycotoxins in animal tissues are not commonly available. We must rely on the detection of mycotoxins in grain or feed to help establish the diagnosis.

Investigation of suspected mycotoxicoses should begin by obtaining thorough histories. Clinical signs are very important because they can be used to select appropriate diagnostic tests to help confirm or refute mycotoxicoses. Investigation of suspected mycotoxicoses should include histopathological examination of tissues from affected animals whenever possible. Specific histopathological lesions may be evidence of mycotoxicoses. If there are no lesions in or evidence of pathology in organs known to be effected by mycotoxins, then likelihood of a mycotoxicosis is reduced.

Confirmation of suspected mycotoxicoses is assisted by either reproducing the clinical disease during a feeding trial using the suspected ration, or by detection of a known mycotoxin in the ration or tissues of animals consuming the ration. Feeding trials are not routinely performed because they are difficult to conduct, expensive, and slow to provide results. Detection of known mycotoxins in feeds is relatively easy with modern analytical chemical methods.

One of the most challenging aspects of diagnosing cases of suspected mycotoxicoses is collecting a feed sample that adequately represents the feed suspected of being contaminated. Mycotoxins are not evenly distributed in feeds, so the contaminated part of the feed may be consumed before disease is evident. Collection of meaningful feed specimens under such conditions is very difficult.

Interpreting the significance of finding mycotoxins present in the ration is difficult. If a mycotoxin is detected in feed, the disease it causes should match the clinical syndrome observed for the case and its concentrations should be sufficient to cause a mycotoxicosis. If not, it is unlikely that the presence of the mycotoxin in the feed is significant.

Treatment of animals suffering from mycotoxicoses usually is supportive and often not very effective. Antidotes for mycotoxins are generally not available. Stopping and preventing further exposure by removing contaminated feed is important.

It is not uncommon for animals to improve after they quit eating feed suspected or known to be contaminated with mycotoxins. Such an occurrence supports the suspicion of the feed as a causal factor, but does not prove that the animals suffered from a mycotoxicosis.

Health effects, clinical signs, lesions and treatment for selected mycotoxicoses.

Aflatoxicosis

Aflatoxicosis is caused by aflatoxins, produced by *Aspergillus flavus* and *Aspergillus parasiticus*. Aflatoxins are commonly found in corn, milo, cottonseed and peanuts. Aflatoxin concentrations in grains produced in Nebraska rarely contain enough aflatoxin to cause acute aflatoxicosis.

There are five important aflatoxins, called aflatoxin B_1, B_2, G_1, G_2, and M_1. Aflatoxin M_1 is a metabolite of aflatoxin B_1 found in milk and urine. It is formed after aflatoxin B_1 enters the body. It is not found in feed. Aflatoxin B_1 is found most frequently and in the highest concentrations in naturally contaminated feed.

Aflatoxin is a liver poison (hepatotoxin) in all species that consume it, however, ruminants tolerate it better than do monogastrics or poultry. It causes liver damage at higher doses and liver cancer at lower doses. Aflatoxin exposure can depress the immune system. It may cause abortions in some instances; however the circumstances necessary for abortions to occur are not well defined.

Clinical Signs of Aflatoxicoses

Acute exposure, all species: Depression, anorexia, reduced gain or milk production, subnormal body temperature.

Chronic exposure, poultry: Decreased growth rate, reduced feed efficiency, steatorrhea (fat in feces), bruising.

Chronic exposure, swine: Anorexia, unthriftiness, slow growth, icterus, mild anemia, ascites, increased susceptibility to infection.

Chronic exposure, cattle: May slow rumen motility for 24 to 48 hours.

Lesions of Aflatoxicosis

Acute exposure: Hemorrhage, ascites.

Chronic exposure: Pale, soft, clay-colored liver, mild anemia, icterus, and ascites.

Histopathological: Hepatocyte degeneration and necrosis; centrilobular hemorrhagic hepatic necrosis, fatty changes and regeneration of hepatocytes; bile duct epithelial proliferation progressing to interlobular fibroplasia and extensive proliferation; Karyomegaly, atypical nuclei, hepatocytic vacuolization, bile retention.

Diagnostic Aids for Aflatoxicosis

Blood workup: Check for anemia, elevated liver enzymes, serum bile acids, albumin:globulin ratio; prothrombin activity.

Tissue or fluid analysis: Aflatoxin M1 present in milk or urine; parent compound may be present in kidney or liver.

Grain or feed analysis: Aflatoxins are most likely to be present in corn, peanuts or cotton seed.

They are not likely to be present in forages or silage at significant concentrations. Dietary aflatoxin concentrations at which performance or clinical effects become noticeable depends upon species and effect. Decreased performance may occur at concentrations as low as 200 ppb in young, sensitive species. Immunity may become impaired at concentrations of about 200 ppb. Hepatic lesions may become noticeable at 200 to 400 ppb. Clinical illness may become obvious at about 400 ppb. Generally, ruminants are most resistant and swine and avian specimens least resistant to adverse effects. Violative residues in milk can occur at concentrations at or near 50 ppb aflatoxin.

Treatment for Aflatoxicosis

Stop exposure: Stop feeding contaminated ration and replace with non-contaminated ration. Supportive treatment: Provide supportive treatment as clinical situation dictates.

Ergot Toxicosis

Ergot toxicosis is a disease caused by the ingestion of ergot alkaloids contained in the sclerotia of *Claviceps* spp. They are commonly found in cereal grains, especially rye. Tall fescue (*Festuca arundinaceae*) may contain the endophytic fungus *Neotyphodium coenophialumin* (*Acremonium coenophialum*), which can also make ergot alkaloids.

Sclerotia are dark brown, brownish-purple or black colored bodies that stick out from the seed heads of infected plants. They are visible to the naked eye and look similar to rodent droppings when removed from the seed heads. They may become quite large, up to an inch in length.

Several different ergot alkaloids may be present in sclerotia. They cause two syndromes: a central nervous system disorder and a peripheral vascular disorder. They can cause agalactia in lactating females.

Ergot alkaloids are potent smooth muscle stimulants. Any organ with smooth muscle in it may be affected, especially arterioles. Uterine contractions may be stimulated.

Clinical Signs of Ergot Toxicosis

Peripheral vascular syndrome: Lameness, swelling of feet and fetlocks; sharply demarcated necrosis of feet, ears or tail. In severe cases, hooves or feet, or tail may slough. Dry gangrene: These effects are due to ischemia resulting from constriction of arterioles in peripheral vascular beds.

Lactating females: Cessation of milk production; agalactia in post-partum females.

Central nervous system syndrome: Hyperexcitability, hypermetria, tremors; heat intolerance in cattle.

Lesions of Ergot Toxicosis

It is described above under clinical signs for peripheral vascular syndrome. Additionally, small and flaccid mammary glands of females in late pregnancy, with no evidence of secretions, are indications of probable agalactia.

Histopathological: Endothelial damage, thrombosis, coagulative necrosis.

Diagnostic Aids for Ergot Toxicosis

Analysis of stomach or rumen content for ergot alkaloids: Detection of ergot alkaloids in stomach or rumen content is evidence of exposure.

Analysis of feed or grains for ergot alkaloids ingested by affected animals. Sclerotia may be visible if the feed has not been ground.

Treatment for Ergot Toxicosis

Stop exposure: Remove contaminated grain or feed from ration. Lactation may commence 5 to 7 days afterwards.

Control secondary infections in limbs suffering from dry gangrene.

Place animals in a warm, clean, stress-free environment.

Fumonisin Toxicosis

Fumonisins are produced by *Fusarium moniliforme* and *F. proliferatum*, and is found primarily in white and yellow corn. There are three kinds, called fumonisins B_1, B_2, and B_3. Fumonisin B_1 is most prevalent in naturally contaminated corn and it is the most toxic.

Horses and pigs are the most sensitive species. Equine leukoencephalomalacia (ELE) is a fatal disease of horses caused by fumonisins. Porcine pulmonary syndrome is the form of the disease in swine. The mechanism of action is believed to be the inhibition of enzymes involved in the production of sphingosine from sphinganine. Sphingosine is an important component of cell membranes, especially for neurons.

Clinical Signs of Fumonisin Toxicosis

Swine: Dyspnea, cyanosis, and weakness, which develop 4-7 days after fumonisin-contaminated feed begins. Death may occur within a few hours of onset of the syndrome.

Horses: Depression, blindness, ataxia, aimless wandering, facial paralysis, which may rapidly progress to coma and death. Death may occur 1 to 7 days after onset of signs.

Ruminants: May develop anorexia and suffer mild weight loss if fumonisin concentrations approach 200 ppm. Few other significant or persistent signs.

Poultry: Appear to be more resistant than other species. Inappetence and skeletal abnormalities may develop at concentrations of 200 - 400 ppm.

Lesions of Fumonisin Toxicosis

Swine: Acute pulmonary edema characterized by marked to massive intralobular pulmonary edema and marked hydrothorax. Lungs are distended and turgid. Thoracic cavity is filled with straw-colored proteinaceous fluid. Microscopically, interstitial and interlobular edema. May include multiple areas of focal pancreatic necrosis and hepatic lesions characterized by disorganized hepatocytes, increased mitotic figures, necrosis of single hepatocytes and mild bile retention. Icterus.

Horses: Leukoencephalomalacia – massive softening and liquefaction of cerebral white matter, ranging from discrete focal areas to large cavitations and inward collapse of the cortical gray matter. Hemorrhage is prominent. Microscopically, liquefaction and proliferation of macrophages in response to necrosis.

Diagnostic Aids for Fumonisin Toxicosis

Blood workup: Evidence of hepatic dysfunction.

Tissue analysis: Sphinganine:sphingosine ratio is increased. Analysis of tissues for sphinganine and sphingosine is not readily available.

Analysis of corn or corn-containing feed for fumonisins: Concentrations in excess of 3 ppm fumonisin may be significant for horses. Concentrations above 5 ppm may be significant for pigs.

Treatment for Fumonisin Toxicosis

Stop exposure: Remove contaminated feed from ration. Because of the long time between consumption of feed and onset of signs, oral detoxification is not recommended.

Supportive treatment: prognosis for horses and pigs suffering from advanced stages of the disease is poor.

Vomitoxin (Deoxynivalenol, DON) Toxicosis

Vomitoxin is produced by *Fusarium roseum* (*F. graminearum*) and *F. moniliforme*. It is found in corn, wheat, barley, milo and occasionally in oats. It is rarely found in hay or forages. *F. Roseum* also produces zearalenone, so DON may also be found with zearalenone.

Vomitoxin is a chemical that belongs to a group of mycotoxins called tricothecenes. There are at least 140 chemicals in that class, including T-2 toxin and diacetoxyscripenol (DAS). Trichothecenes other than vomitoxin are rarely, if ever, found in grain grown in Nebraska.

Vomitoxin is not very toxic, but it is associated with feed refusal and decreased feed consumption, which can affect animal performance. Concentrations ranging from 5 to 10 ppm are associated with vomiting in pigs, hence its name. Thresholds for decreased feed intake are about 1 ppm in swine and 10 to 20 ppm in ruminants.

The mechanism by which vomitoxin acts has not been elucidated. Other trichothecenes inhibit protein and nucleic acid synthesis.

Cattle are very resistant to the effects of vomitoxin. Pigs are more sensitive. There have been reports of health effects in dogs from pet foods contaminated with vomitoxin-containing grains.

Clinical Signs of Vomitoxin Toxicosis

Swine, dogs, cats – feed refusal, vomiting; cattle – usually none, however some reports of feed refusal may be found in the scientific literature; poultry – usually none.

Lesions of Vomitoxin Toxicosis

No gross or histopathological lesions have been reported in animals consuming vomitoxin-contaminated feed.

Diagnostic Aids for Vomitoxin Toxicosis

Analysis of grains or feeds: Forages are seldom, if ever, contaminated with vomitoxin.

Analysis of tissues from affected animals: Not available.

Treatment for Vomitoxin Toxicosis

Remove vomitoxin-contaminated grain/feed from ration.

Zearalenone Toxicosis

Zearalenone is produced by *Fusarium roseum* (*F. graminearum*) and *F. moniliforme*. It is found in corn, wheat, barley, milo and occasionally in oats. F. Roseum also produces vomitoxin (deoxynivalenol, DON), so vomitoxin may also be found with zearalenone.

Zearalenone is a chemical that can act similarly to the female sex hormone estrogen. Excessive exposure does not cause death or abortions, but it can disrupt the estrus cycle in females, cause infertility and feminization in males, and precocious puberty in sexually immature females. Zearalenone content typically found in Nebraska grains is usually not enough to adversely affect animals, but unusual environmental conditions during the growing season, or insufficiently dried grain put up for storage may increase zearalenone production.

Clinical Signs of Zearalenone Toxicosis

Clinical signs vary with species, sex and age of the animal.

Swine, sexually immature gilts: Behavioral estrus, swollen and edematous vulva, enlarged mammary glands, tenesmus (spasmodic contraction of anal or bladder sphincter), sometimes vaginal or rectal prolapse; clinical signs appear 2-7 days after exposure begins and subsides 4 to 10 days after exposure ends.

Swine, mature sows: Exposure early in estrus cycle – suppression of ovulation and signs of estrus that are severe and prolonged; exposure mid-cycle – pseudopregnancy, anestrus which may persist for 40 to 60 days after exposure stops.

Swine, castrated boars: Enlarged prepuce and nipples.

Swine, immature boars: Reduced libido, retarded testicular development.

Swine, mature boars: Not effected unless dietary concentrations reach 200 ppm or higher. Such concentrations are rarely encountered in U.S. grains.

Lesions of Zearalenone Toxicosis

Lesions are present only in the reproductive system.

Prepubertal gilts: Swollen and edematous vulva; enlarged mammary glands; enlarged, hypertrophic and edematous uterus. Histopathologically, uterine and vaginal metaplasia and follicular atresia.

Mature sows: Retained and functional corpora lutea with anestrus. Mammary alveolar development and ductular sqamous metaplasia.

Diagnostic Aids for Zearalenone Toxicosis

Blood workup: Serum analysis for estrogen can help rule out an organic hormonal problem.

Tissue or fluid analysis: Not available.

Feed or grain analysis: Since clinical effects are delayed several days after ingestion, feed analysis may be of limited value. A specimen collected after the problem is noticed may not contain detectable amounts of zearalenone. Planned retention and dating of feed specimens aids in the identification of zearalenone-contaminated feed.

Differential Considerations for Zearalenone Toxicosis

Other estrogenic chemicals from plants (phyto estrogens) or other sources could also produce some of the signs of zearalenone toxicosis. An expensive, but possibly valuable estrogenic assay of feed is available to help assess estrogenic activity of the feed. That assay detects any chemical with estrogenic activity that might be present in the feed.

Treatment for Zearalenone Toxicosis

Stop exposure: Remove contaminated feed and replace with uncontaminated feed. Signs may persist for several days afterwards.

Decrease zearalenone absorption: Activated charcoal may help limit absorption of ingested zearalenone by individual animals. Several commercially available feed additives are advertized to bind zearalenone and help prevent excessive exposure. The efficacy of such additives may not have been adequately assessed. Thoroughly assess the evidence offered by manufacturers before using them. Such use may require approval by federal regulatory agencies before it can be used legally.

Fungal Infections in Animals

The past few decades has witnessed medical, veterinary and ecological excrescence of fungal diseases with a dramatic increase coupled with a myriad of pathognomonic manifestations in both animals and humans. To worsen the situation, climate change induced/related emergence of fungal infections is also evident irrespective of geographical region with new host spectrum/species. The emergence of Chytrid fungus *Batrachochytrium dendrobatidis* among amphibian population is the classic example in this regard which contributes extinctions of several frog species. Coral reef depletion due to *Aspergillus sydowii*, mass mortalities of turtle by *Fusarium solani* and white nose syndrome due to *Pseudogymnoascus (Geomyces) destructans* in bats are other major emerging fungal diseases worldwide in animals with crippling impacts. In humans, rise of immunocompromised people opens new avenues for fungal diseases which are further complicated by diabetes and currently the COVID-19 complications. According to the Global Action Fund for Fungal Infections (GAFFI), over 300 million people of all ages suffer from serious fungal diseases every year, resulting in over 13,50,000 deaths globally.

The post-COVID-19 fungal infections have wreaked havoc among public health authorities as more and more cases are reporting incessantly from several countries. The cascade of immunological responses during COVID-19 like pulmonary epithelial damage, immunological malignancies, highly permissive inflammatory environment all create a conducive environment for fungi to invade and cause infection. The global emergence of antifungal resistance by fungal pathogens has made the treatment more challenging and perplexed. The climate change connections in the emergence of fungal diseases are also well reported which is well connected with global warming. To conclude, fungi, the neglected groups of organisms are now parading towards the main stage with ruinous clinical manifestations and incidence rates with unimaginable perturbations in public health arena. Thus, conglomerated efforts and actions are the need of the hour to cop up with the diseases due to fungi in both animals and humans.

Fungus Infection in an Animal

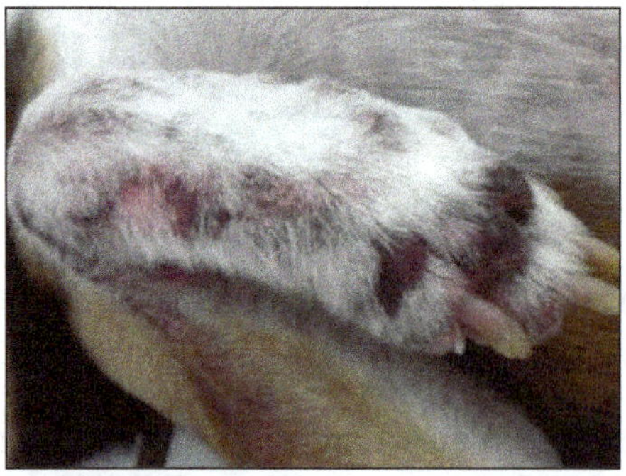

Fungal infection on right forelimb of dog.

Fungi are ubiquitous organisms that live in the soil and in the environment. They often perform important ecological roles such as helping to break down organic debris (rotting food, stool or plant material). Most infections can be acquired by ingestion, inhalation, or even through the skin (transdermally). Fungal infections may reach the brain and spinal cord by direct spread from an adjacent infection occurring in the nasal cavity, sinuses, outer ear, Eustachian tube, and middle/inner ear. Infection may also be transmitted via a migrating foreign body. Fungal infections of the central nervous system (CNS) in dogs and cats are uncommon; however, when they do occur, they can be devastating and particularly aggressive. Fungal infection is more likely in young to middle-aged dogs and cats (1-7 years). Several types of fungi can invade the CNS including *Cryptococcus*, *Coccidioides*, *Blastomyces*, *Histoplasma*, and *Aspergillus* species. Opportunistic fungi, such as *Aspergillus* and *Cryptococcus,* usually require a debilitated or immunosuppressed host to establish infection; however, all strains are capable of producing a primary infection despite this compromised state. *Cryptococcus neoformans* is the most common fungal organism associated with infection of the CNS in dogs and cats.

Clinical Signs

Clinical signs are dependent on the lesion location (whether in the brain, spinal cord or both) and severity of the infection. These signs are often multifocal or diffuse in nature making diagnosis somewhat difficult. Neurological signs may reflect brain involvement (i.e. seizures, depression, disorientation, circling, anisocoria, pupillary dilation, and central blindness), spinal cord involvement, (ataxia, pelvic limb paresis, paraplegia, and spinal hyperesthesia) or a combination of these signs. Deficits of one or several cranial nerves are often present. Patients can show evidence of concurrent systemic disease with signs such as skin lesions, nasal/frontal sinus swelling or drainage, fever, weight loss, inflammation of the iris of the eye, blindness, lameness, enlarged lymph nodes, coughing, and wheezing. While neurologic dysfunction may be acute in onset and rapidly progressive, fungal infection of the CNS is often characterized by a slow progression over weeks to months with a period of non-specific illness (lethargy or anorexia) beforehand. Thus, fungal disease can be all too easily missed until it has spread into vital areas of the body and become overwhelming and potentially fatal.

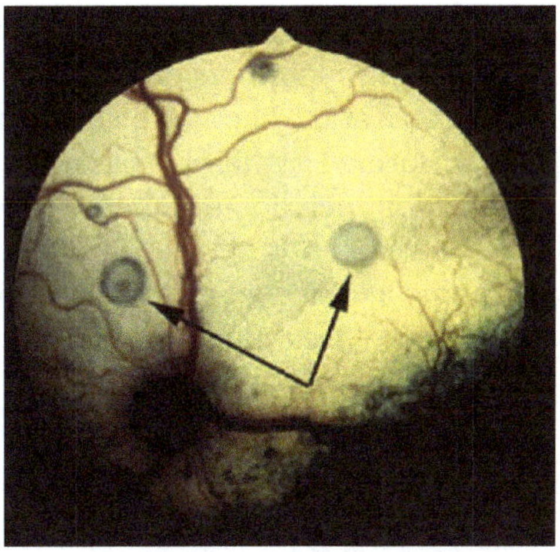

Retinal cryptococcosis in cat eye.

Diagnosis

Diagnosis of a fungal infection within the CNS is ultimately based on direct visualization of the organism. Routine laboratory tests are often normal, although there may be evidence of chronic disease such as anemia. Fungal elements are occasionally identified on urinalysis. Thoracic radiographs may show evidence of a fungal disease process by either a diffuse or nodular interstitial lung pattern with those pathogens which can infect the respiratory system. Magnetic resonance imaging (MRI) can be used and is likely to show lesions that strongly contrast enhance. Both focal lesions, such as a fungal granuloma, and more diffuse disease processes, such as meningitis, can be visualized on MRI. These findings are useful for therapeutic decisions and grading severity of the infection. Fungal serology can also be used whenever direct visualization is not possible or to support a diagnosis and is easily done in routine clinical practice. With serology, a blood sample is collected and serum sent to specialized laboratory in order to assess for antibodies against specific fungal antigens. For Cryptococcus, serum is directly tested for detection of the antigen itself.

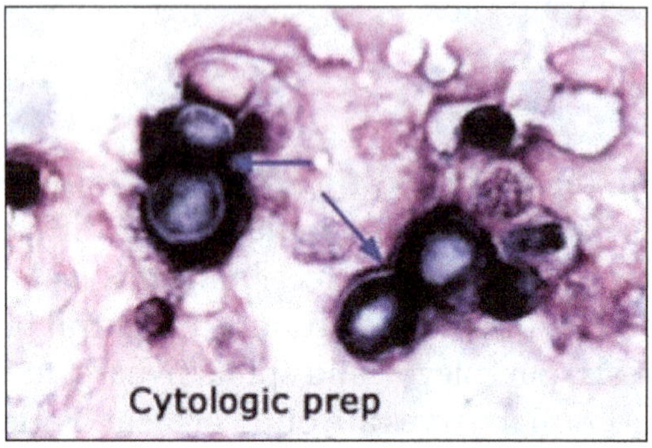

Blastomyces on cytology.

Definitive diagnosis is made via cytology, biopsy, or culture of an affected organ or cerebrospinal fluid (CSF). Cytology is performed either by impression smears or fine needle aspirate and fungal hyphae or spores may be visualized under the microscope. If surgery is pursued, a portion of the specimen can be obtained by surgical biopsy and submitted for histopathology. This allows for a larger sample to be collected compared to cytological collection techniques. Cultures are frequently used in suspected fungal cases but have the drawback of delayed results while waiting for the pathogen to grow in the laboratory. In these cases, treatment is usually begun before confirming the diagnosis so that more life threatening symptoms do not develop. Cerebrospinal fluid is collected from the cerebellomedullary cistern at the back of the head or the subarachnoid space in the lumbar region and should only be performed by highly trained veterinary professionals. Typical abnormalities seen that support infection include an increased protein content, increased numbers of white cells as well as the presence of eosinophils. On CSF cytology, fungal organisms may be visible. Practitioners should combine a variety of the available tests to confirm the presence of a pathogen and decide on the best course of treatment.

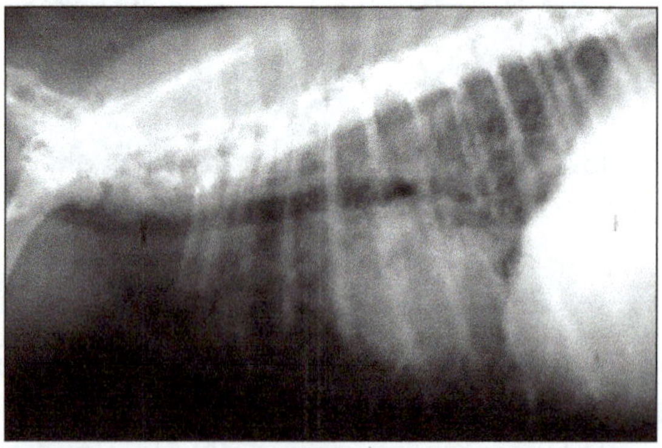

Coccidioidomycosis in thoracic radiograph.

Treatment

Fungal infections within the CNS of animals can be difficult to treat for a host of reasons. While antifungal therapy is considered the primary treatment for fungal infections, most antifungal agents do not adequately cross the blood-brainbarrier (BBB). One of the few antifungal drugs that will cross the BBB is fluconazole. It constitutes the first line course of treatment because high drug concentrations can be achieved in the CNS. Fluconazole has the added benefit of being available in a variety of formulations; however, higher doses are usually needed for CNS disease. Voriconazole is especially effective against several fungal species, but reserved for when other azole fungal agents fail. It is very expensive and can lead to client frustration and non-compliance. Amphotericin B is especially toxic to the kidneys and should only be used in severe cases as some renal damage is possible following treatment. Itraconazole has the fewest side effects of all the azole agents, but does not reach minimum inhibitory concentrations in the cerebrospinal fluid.

Unfortunately, in some cases, antifungal medications by themselves are not enough to completely treat infection. Surgical removal/debulking of intracranial granulomas may be indicated depending on the size, location, and the presence of any potential fatal complications (ie. increased intracranial pressure, edema). Surgical intervention comes with significant cost to the client, risk to the patient, and significant recovery time which should be discussed at length before pursuing this treatment route. While corticosteroids are frequently utilized to reduce secondary inflammation and cerebral edema, their use is controversial and usually contraindicated in fungal infections due to immunosuppression. If corticosteroids are used, they should be used judiciously and short term. Lastly, it is not uncommon for fungal organisms to lie dormant in the CNS and return after withdrawal of antifungal therapy. As a result, clients need to be prepared emotionally and financially for long-term treatment, sometimes greater than the period of a year, even after clinical signs of the disease appear to be gone. The decision regarding when to discontinue antifungal therapy should be based on presence of clinical signs, repeat CSF results, and CSF/serum titers for the organism.

Superficial Candidiasis

Superficial candidiasis includes infections of cutaneous or mucocutaneous tissues. *Candida albicans* is the causative agent in the majority of infections. Other Candida species that can cause the superficial infections include *C. tropicalis, C. glabrata, C. parapsilosis, C. stellatoidea, C. dubliniensis*, and *C. krusei*. Superficial candidiasis can be acute, chronic, or recurrent. Candida spp. and *C. albicans*, in particular, are ubiquitous dimorphic fungal organisms that are part of the normal microflora of healthy individuals. However, they are also opportunistic pathogens that can quickly transform from the harmless mucosal commensal to a highly pathogenic organism of the same tissues with significant morbidity and even mortality under the appropriate conditions.

Superficial candidiasis can include skin, oropharyngeal, gastrointestinal, vaginal, and conjunctival tissue infections. Cutaneous candidiasis usually occurs as erythematous patches on the thigh and buttocks, or as superficial infections of the hands in individuals who routinely wear plastic gloves. Mucocutaneous infections may be chronic and/or recurrent and one particular form is classified as the disorder known as chronic mucocutaneous candidiasis (CMC). These infections affect a variety of mucosal tissues, skin, and nails. Oropharyngeal candidiasis (OPC) involves infections of the buccal mucosa, gingiva, and tongue. The infections can be atrophic with erythematous lesions or pseudomembranous (thrush) with characteristic white lesions.

Esophagitis is the most common form of gastrointestinal candidiasis. It is extremely painful and can promote wasting because of the difficulty with swallowing. The second most common site of gastrointestinal candidiasis is the stomach. Vaginitis involves infections of the vaginal lumen and often the vulva as well. An estimated 75 percent of all women will experience an episode of acute vulvovaginal candidiasis (VVC) in their lifetime with 5–10 percent succumbing to recurrent VVC (RVVC). Conjunctivitis caused by *C. albicans* infects the mucous membranes of the eye, while keratitis affects the cornea. Table summarizes the common superficial *Candida* infections.

Host defense mechanisms that protect against *C. albicans* infections include innate resistance and acquired immunity. The relative contributions of these two systems, however, differ depending upon the site at which *C. albicans* enters the host. Innate host defenses (i.e. polymorphonuclear leukocytes, macrophages) are heavily involved in protecting the systemic circulation, antibodies (i.e. IgA, IgG) appear to play a role at both systemic and mucosal sites, and cell-mediated immunity (CMI) (i.e. T cells, relevant cytokines) protects primarily mucosal tissues. With regard to mucosal tissues, while historically there was no distinction between different anatomic sites, there is now increasing evidence that 'not all mucosal tissues are created equal' relative to protective host defenses. Accordingly, current data show roles for several types of host responses at any one site, albeit at different levels of priority with respect to their protective capacity. This review covers the epidemiology of each superficial infection, properties of *C. albicans* as a commensal of the gastrointestinal and genitourinary tracts, properties of *C. albicans* as a pathogen causing superficial infections, and host defenses critical to protection against and susceptibility to superficial candidiasis at the various anatomic sites.

Table: Common superficial Candida infections.

Cutaneous
Mucocutaneous
Oropharyngeal
Gastrointestinal: stomach; esophageal
Vaginal
Conjunctival/keratitis

Oropharyngeal Candidiasis (OPC)

OPC involves infections of the hard and soft palate, tongue, buccal mucosa, and floor of the mouth. It presents as reddened patches (erythematous) or white curd-like lesions (pseudomembranous). Chewing and swallowing can be difficult under these conditions. Infections can be acute or recurrent, and are common in immunocompromised patients especially those infected with the human immunodeficiency virus (HIV). OPC is also a common manifestation of CMC (reviewed in Odds 1988a) and occurs in patients with lymphoma, those undergoing steroid therapy, and in transplant recipients. Although OPC will occur under several immunocompromising conditions, it appears to be much more common in HIV-infected persons than under any other condition. In fact, OPC is often one of the first clinical signs of underlying HIV infection and will occur in 50–95 percent of all HIV-positive persons sometime during their progression to full-blown acquired immunodeficiency syndrome (AIDS). Thus, it is possible that a link between HIV and OPC is present that enhances susceptibility to OPC. Interestingly, highly active antiretroviral therapy (HAART) has reduced the incidence of OPC. This is postulated to be due both to increased immune responsiveness as well as the action of the protease inhibitors in HAART on the secretory aspartyl proteases (SAP), an important virulence factor of *C. albicans*.

Gastrointestinal Candidiasis

For the purposes of the discussion at hand, gastrointestinal (GI) candidiasis will be defined as infections of the esophagus, stomach, and small and large intestines. GI candidiasis is not easily recognized clinically but does occur in cancer patients who are heavily immunosuppressed and patients receiving antibiotic prophylaxis. Esophagitis is the most common form of gastrointestinal candidiasis that occurs in later stages of immunosuppression and is considered an AIDS-defining illness. It is extremely painful and can promote wasting because of the difficulty with swallowing. White plaques are usually observed similar to thrush. Complications include bleeding and perforation. Diagnosis is made on appearance of ulcers and erosions on the esophagus, and may need to be confirmed by endoscopy and biopsy of the affected site. The second most common site of GI candidiasis is the stomach where symptoms of gastritis occur. GI candidiasis is sometimes difficult to diagnose due to the lack of specific symptoms and the lack of the ability to differentiate between infectious and commensal *C. albicans*.

Vaginal Candidiasis

Vulvovaginal candidiasis (VVC) affects a significant number of women predominantly in their reproductive years. An estimated 75 percent of all women will experience an episode of acute VVC in their lifetime with another 5–10 percent succumbing to RVVC. Vaginitis involves infections of the vaginal lumen and often the vulva as well. Symptoms include burning, itching, soreness, an abnormal discharge, and dyspareunia. Signs include vaginal and vulvar erythema and edema. Acute VVC has several known predisposing factors including antibiotic and oral contraceptive usage, hormone replacement therapy, pregnancy, uncontrolled diabetes mellitus, and immunosuppressive therapy. RVVC is multifactorial in etiology, but is usually defined as idiopathic with no known predisposing factors in the majority of those affected. In women with RVVC, antifungal therapy is highly effective for individual symptomatic attacks, but does not prevent subsequent recurrence. There is little evidence that resistance to antifungal drugs plays a role in the pathogenesis of RVVC. Instead, susceptibility to RVVC is postulated to be immune-based in that these otherwise healthy women experience repeated symptomatic episodes as a result of some immunological dysfunction or deficiency. Furthermore, it is postulated that recurrences are a result of relapse rather than reinfection since strain types of *C. albicans* tend to remain the same in women for multiple recurrences over several years. This is consistent with the fact that antifungal drugs are static rather than cidal and as such; do not completely eliminate the organisms.

Pityriasis Versicolor

Pityriasis versicolor is a common yeast infection of the skin, in which flaky discoloured patches appear on the chest and back.

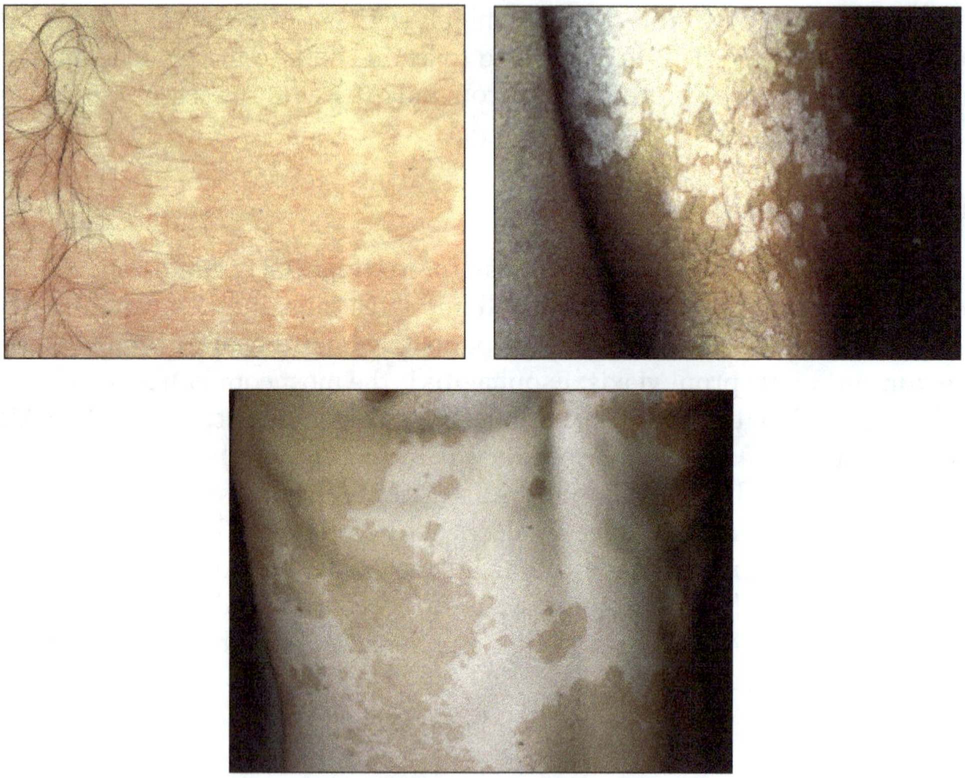

Pityriasis versicolor.

The term pityriasis is used to describe skin conditions in which the scale appears similar to bran. The multiple colours of pityriasis versicolor give rise to the second part of the name, versicolor. Pityriasis versicolor is sometimes called tinea versicolor, although the term tinea should strictly be used for dermatophyte fungus infections.

Susceptible to Pityriasis Versicolor

Pityriasis versicolor most frequently affects young adults and is slightly more common in men than in women. It can also affect children, adolescents, and older adults.

Pityriasis versicolor is more common in hot, humid climates than in cool, dry climates. It often affects people who perspire heavily. It may clear in the winter months and recur each summer.

Although it is not considered infectious in the conventional sense, pityriasis versicolor sometimes affects more than one member of a family.

Cause of Pityriasis Versicolor

Pityriasis versicolor is caused by mycelial growth of fungi of the genus *Malassezia*.

Malassezia are part of the normal skin microbiota (microorganisms found on normal skin). They are dependent on lipid for survival. Fourteen different species of malassezia have been identified. The most common species cultured from pityriasis versicolor are *M. globosa*, *M. restricta* and *M. sympodialis*.

Usually malassezia grow sparsely in the seborrhoeic areas (scalp, face and chest) without causing a rash. It is not known why they sometimes grow more actively on the skin surface to form pityriasis versicolor. One theory implicates a tryptophan-dependent metabolic pathway.

The yeasts induce enlarged melanosomes (pigment granules) within basal melanocytes in the brown type of pityriasis versicolor. It is easier to demonstrate the yeasts in scrapings taken from this type of pityriasis versicolor than in those taken from the white type.

The white or hypopigmented type of pityriasis versicolor is thought to be due to a chemical produced by malassezia that diffuses into the epidermis and impairs the function of the melanocytes.

The pink type of pityriasis versicolor is mildly inflamed, due to dermatiits induced by malassezia or its metabolites.

Clinical Features of Pityriasis Versicolor

Pityriasis versicolor affects the trunk, neck, and/or arms, and is uncommon on other parts of the body. The patches may be coppery brown, paler than surrounding skin, or pink. Pale patches may be more common in darker skin; this appearance is known as pityriasis versicolor alba. Sometimes the patches start scaly and brown, and then resolve through a non-scaly and white stage.

Pityriasis versicolor is usually asymptomatic, but in some people it is mildly itchy.

In general, pale or dark patches due to pityriasis versicolor do not tend to be more or less prone to sunburn than surrounding skin.

Hyperpigmented, hypopigmented, and pink pityriasis versicolor are usually seen as distinct variants but may sometimes co-exist. Pink pityriasis versicolor may also co-exist with seborrhoeic dermatitis as both are associated with malassezia overgrowth.

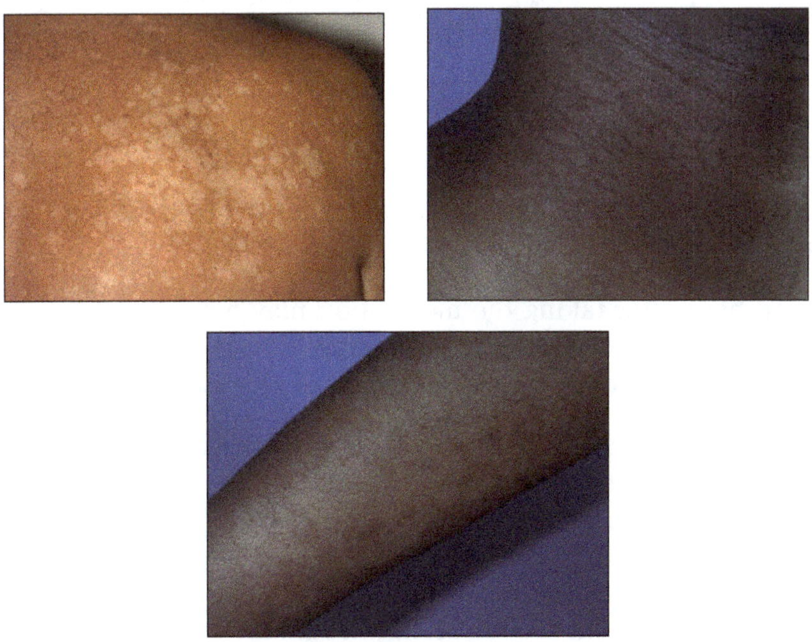

Pityriasis versicolor.

Diagnosis of Pityriasis Versicolor

Pityriasis versicolor is usually diagnosed clinically. The following tests may be useful.

- Wood lamp (black light) examination — yellow-green fluorescence may be observed in affected areas.
- Dermoscopy of pityriasis versicolor — pallor, background faint pigment network, and scale.
- Microscopy of a skin scraping (using potassium hydroxide (KOH) to remove skin cells) — hyphae and yeast cells that resemble spaghetti and meatballs.
- Fungal culture — this is usually reported to be negative, as it is quite difficult to persuade the yeasts to grow in a laboratory.
- Skin biopsy — fungal elements may be seen within the outer cells of the skin (stratum corneum) on histopathology. Special stains may be required.

Treatment of Pityriasis Versicolor

Topical Measures

Mild pityriasis versicolor is treated with topical antifungal agents.

- Selenium sulfide shampoo.
- Topical azole cream/shampoo (econazole, ketoconazole).
- Terbinafine gel.

The medicine should be applied widely to the skin from the jawline down and left on the skin for 5-15 minutes before rinsing off in the shower. This should be done daily for one week then weekly for one month.

Systemic Measures

Oral antifungal agents, itraconazole and fluconazole, are used to treat pityriasis versicolor when extensive or if topical agents have failed.

Vigorous exercise an hour after taking the medication may help sweat it onto the skin surface, where it can effectively eradicate the yeast. Bathing should be avoided for a few hours. A few days' treatment will clear many cases of pityriasis long term, or at least for several months.

Oral terbinafine, an antifungal agent used to treat dermatophyte infections, is not effective for yeast infections such as pityriasis versicolor.

Preventative Measures

Reapplication of a topical treatment such as selenium sulfide shampoo every month once the rash has cleared will usually prevent recurrence.

Prevention and Control of Fungal Infections

Reports of human infections with environmental fungi are on the increase throughout the world. Many of these reports describe infections caused by new agents, as well as by traditional agents with new virulence factors or new mechanisms of infection. Fungal infections historically have been under recognized and difficult to detect, and treatment options are poor.

The reasons for their emergence are likely multifactorial. The advent of medical progress—including the wide use of medical hardware, such as central lines; successful management of immunosuppression in patients with transplanted organs; and immunomodulatory agents for treating underlying diseases from cancer to rheumatoid arthritis—has contributed to the increase in fungal infections in immunocompromised hosts. Risk factors such as changes in land use, seasonal migration, international travel, extreme weather, and natural disasters, and the use of azole antifungal agents in large-scale agriculture are believed to underlie many of the increases in community-acquired fungal infections.

Because fungal infections are frequently under recognized and difficult to detect, one of the largest gaps in our understanding of their epidemiology is determining the incidence of disease. In an article in this issue of Emerging Infectious Diseases, Sondermeyer et al. document the incidence and cost of hospitalizations in California caused by Valley fever (coccidioidomycosis), a fungal infection endemic to the southwestern United States and parts of Latin America. This article reports that during 2000–2011, there were >25,000 Valley fever–associated hospitalizations in California and >$2 billion in hospital costs. The rate of hospitalizations increased over the study period from 2.3 to 5.0 cases/100,000 population, a finding that supports other recent publications documenting the increasing incidence of Valley fever in the United States. Although the reasons for this increase are not well understood, the practical effect of this increasing incidence has been seen in many settings, including the California state prison system. Recently, a federal court ordered the prison system to move prisoners believed to be at high risk for Valley fever (including Blacks, persons >55 years of age, and persons with preexisting diabetes) out of 2 prisons in the San Joaquin Valley, which is the region in California to which coccidioidomycosis is endemic.

Fungal diseases also appear to be emerging beyond their traditionally described borders for reasons that are not entirely understood. One article in this issue reports the incidence of *Cryptococcus gattii* disease, once believed to be restricted to tropical regions, but which is now found in locations as disparate as Vancouver Island, Canada and parts of the southeastern United States. Although this organism is genetically related to *C. neoformans*, a cause of meningitis in HIV-infected persons, *C. gattii* is frequently associated with a different spectrum of disease, prominently pneumonia. In another article in this issue, Nucci et al. report an increase in incidence of community-associated *Fusarium* spp. infections in a cancer ward in Brazil. In this study, *Fusarium* spp. caused an increase in invasive infections, which usually started as skin or nail infections, in immunocompetent and immunosuppressed patients. Although the root cause was not determined, speculation has centered on changes in land use patterns and agricultural practices in Brazil. Also in this issue, a novel agent of fungemia, *Candida auris*, is reported as having been detected in India. All isolates reported in this article were resistant to the antifungal agent fluconazole, which is concerning because fluconazole is frequently the first-line treatment for invasive *Candida* spp. infections in many countries. Finally, an article by Fong et al. provides serologic evidence that *Pneumocystis jirovecii* may be transmitted between patients and providers in the health care setting, a finding that could affect future infection control policies.

Because most invasive fungal infections have high mortality rates, reducing the incidence of these diseases often relies on rapid and specific diagnostics, effective antifungal drugs, novel immunotherapeutic strategies, and adherence to infection control and sterility practices. Recently, we have seen examples of successes and failures in this area. In regions with high HIV prevalence, use of novel lateral-flow diagnostic tests for cryptococcal disease has opened the door to systematic screening and point-of-care testing in asymptomatic persons with low CD4 cell counts and may result in reduction of deaths caused by this disease. Conversely, recent contamination of a widely distributed injectable steroid medication with fungal organisms, particularly the black mold *Exserohilum rostratum*, caused the largest health care–associated outbreak in the United States; as of July 1, 2013, there have been 749 cases of meningitis and related infections among persons in 20 states and 61 deaths. Swift public health actions, including notification of patients and providers, led to rapid clinical assessments and institution of antifungal therapy among infected persons, thereby reducing the mortality rate and effects of this disease.

Broader control of fungal exposures in the community can also be improved by awareness, especially education regarding high-risk practices and activities. Outbreaks of histoplasmosis linked to construction and cleaning activities in places contaminated with bird or bat guano have led to production of educational materials describing how risk can be mitigated. Furthermore, recent advances in whole-genome sequencing are being explored to suggest novel vaccine and diagnostic targets for the agent of Valley fever.

Fungal infections remain serious and underappreciated causes of illness and death. Much can be done to prevent the consequences of these infections, although environmental exposure to these agents may not be entirely avoidable in the community. Continued public health efforts toward defining, characterizing, and tracking the emergence of fungal infections can help to focus studies on priority infections and settings. Future translational research is urgently needed to develop novel diagnostics, vaccines, and treatments as more is learned about the pathogenesis of fungal infections and the biology of fungal agents.

Diagnosis and Treatment of Fungal Infections

The definitive diagnosis of any fungal infection requires histopathologic identification of the fungus invading tissue and accompanying evidence of an inflammatory response. The identification of an inflammatory response has been especially important with regard to *Aspergillus* infection. *Aspergillus* is ubiquitous and can float in the air onto biopsy material. Therefore, in rare but important instances, this fungus is an ex vivo contaminant during processing of a specimen for microscopy, with a consequent incorrect diagnosis. The stains most commonly used to identify fungi are periodic acid–Schiff and Gomori methenamine silver. *Candida*, unlike other fungi, is visible on gram-stained tissue smears. Hematoxylin and eosin stain is not sufficient to identify *Candida* in tissue specimens. When positive, an India ink preparation of cerebrospinal fluid (CSF) is diagnostic for cryptococcosis. Most laboratories now use calcofluor white staining coupled with fluorescent microscopy to identify fungi in fluid specimens. Matrix-assisted laser desorption ionization–time of flight mass spectometry (MALDI-TOF MS) will likely be used extensively for detection and speciation in the future. Point-of-care, lateral-flow testing techniques are being developed for many fungal infections.

Extensive investigations of the diagnosis of deep organ fungal infections have yielded a variety of tests with different degrees of specificity and sensitivity. The most reliable tests are the detection of antibody to *Coccidioides immitis* in serum and CSF; of *Histoplasma capsulatum* antigen in urine, serum, and CSF; and of cryptococcal polysaccharide antigen in serum and CSF. Commercially available antibody detection systems can now be used for blastomycosis, histoplasmosis, cryptococcosis, aspergillosis, and β-glucan detection. These tests have a general sensitivity and specificity of 90%; however, because of variability among laboratories, testing on multiple occasions is advisable. The test for galactomannan has been used extensively in Europe and is now approved in the United States for diagnosis of aspergillosis. Sources of concern regarding galactomannan are the incidence of false-negative results and the need for multiple serial tests to reduce this incidence. This test is most useful when applied to bronchoalveolar lavage fluid. The β-glucan test for *Candida* is also under evaluation but, like the galactomannan test, requires additional validation; this test has a negative predictive value of ~90%. Both of these tests are being used with increasing frequency, especially for guiding the timing of initiation and the duration of therapy and for following principles of antimicrobial stewardship. One of the most useful applications of these non-culture-based tests has been the detection of *Histoplasma* antigens in serum and urine. T2 magnetic resonance is also being extensively evaluated for *Candida* and other organisms. It has been approved by the U.S. Food and Drug Administration (FDA) for detection of *Candida* in serum. Numerous polymerase chain reaction assays to detect antigens are in the developmental stages, as are nucleic acid hybridization techniques; currently, these tests are not widely available.

Of the fungal organisms, *Candida* is by far the most frequently recovered from blood. Although *Candida* species can be detected with any of the automated blood culture systems widely used at present, the lysis–centrifugation technique increases the sensitivity of blood cultures for *Candida* and for less common organisms (e.g., *H. capsulatum*). Lysis–centrifugation should be used when disseminated fungal infection is suspected.

Except in the cases of coccidioidomycosis, cryptococcosis, and histoplasmosis, there are no fully validated and widely used tests for serodiagnosis of disseminated fungal infection. Skin tests for the endemic mycoses are no longer available.

This discussion is intended as a brief overview of general strategies for the use of antifungal agents in the treatment of fungal infections. Regimens, schedules, and choices are detailed in the chapters on specific mycoses that follow in this section. The doses cited here are standard doses for adults with invasive infection.

Since fungal organisms are eukaryotic cells that contain most of the same organelles (with many of the same physiologic functions) as human cells, the identification of drugs that selectively kill or inhibit fungi, but are not toxic to human cells, has been highly problematic. Far fewer antifungal than antibacterial agents have been introduced into clinical medicine.

Chapter 3

Fungal Infections of the Skin and Nails

Oral Thrush/Oropharyngeal Candidiasis

Thrush is a kind of yeast infection that's common in the mouths of babies and toddlers. It's rarely serious but can be passed between babies and breastfeeding mothers.

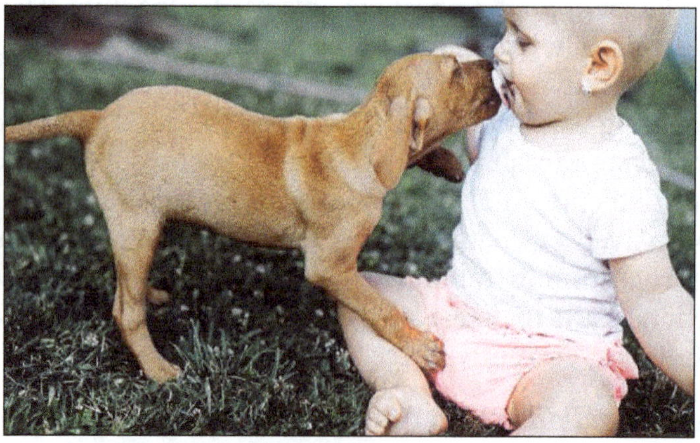

It's normal for a small amount of fungus to live in your mouth. But in some cases, the fungus may rapidly multiply and lead to a yeast infection.

Oral thrush happens when this type of yeast infection develops inside your mouth. It's also known as oral candidiasis, oropharyngeal candidiasis, or simply thrush.

Oral thrush most often occurs in infants and toddlers. It causes white or yellowish lesions or spots to form on the inner cheeks, tongue, gums, lips, and roof of the mouth. Those spots usually go away with treatment.

The infection is typically mild and rarely causes serious problems. It's often easily treated. But in people with weakened immune systems, it can spread to other parts of the body and cause potentially serious complications.

Symptoms of Oral Thrush

In its early stages, oral thrush may not cause any symptoms. But as the infection gets worse, one or more of the following symptoms may develop:

- White or yellow spots on your inner cheeks, tongue, tonsils, gums, or lips.

- Slight bleeding if the spots are scraped.
- Soreness or burning in your mouth.
- A cotton-like sensation in your mouth.
- Dry, cracked skin at the corners of your mouth.
- Difficulty swallowing.
- A bad taste in your mouth.
- A loss of taste.
- Redness, irritation, and pain under dentures (denture stomatitis).

In some cases, oral thrush can affect your esophagus, though this is uncommon. The same fungus that causes oral thrush can also cause yeast infections in other parts of your body. There are also various other symptoms of oral thrush and other types of yeast infections.

Causes of Oral Thrush

Oral thrush and other yeast infections are caused by an overgrowth of the fungus *Candida albicans (C. albicans).*

It's normal for a small amount of *C. albicans* to live in your mouth, without causing harm. When your immune system is working properly, beneficial bacteria in your body help keep *C. albicans* under control.

But if your immune system is compromised or the balance of microorganisms in your body is disrupted, the fungus can grow out of control.

You may develop an overgrowth of *C. albicans* that causes oral thrush if you take certain medications that reduce the number of friendly microorganisms in your body, such as antibiotics.

Cancer treatments, including chemotherapy and radiation therapy, can also damage or kill healthy cells. This makes you more susceptible to oral thrush and other infections.

Conditions that weaken your immune system, such as leukemia and HIV, also increase the risk of developing oral thrush. Oral thrush is a common opportunistic infection in people with HIV.

Diabetes can contribute to oral thrush as well. Uncontrolled diabetes weakens your immune system and causes high blood sugar levels. This creates favorable conditions for *C. albicans* to grow.

Spreading of Oral Thrush

If you have oral thrush, it's possible to pass the fungus that causes this condition on to someone else if you kiss them. In some cases, that person might develop oral thrush.

The fungus that causes oral thrush also causes yeast infections in other body parts. It's possible for you to pass the fungus from one part of your body to another part of someone else's body.

If you have oral thrush, a vaginal yeast infection, or a penile yeast infection, you can potentially pass the fungus to your partner through vaginal sex, anal sex, or oral sex.

If you're pregnant and you have a vaginal yeast infection, you can potentially pass the fungus to your baby during delivery.

If you have a breast yeast infection or nipple yeast infection, you can pass the fungus to your baby while breastfeeding. Your baby can also transmit the fungus to you if they breastfeed when they have oral thrush.

When *C. albicans* is passed from one person to another, it doesn't always cause oral thrush or other types of yeast infection.

Also, because *C. albicans* is so common in our environment, developing a yeast infection does not mean you necessarily caught it from someone else. Learn about some of the factors that can raise your risk of developing an infection when someone passes this fungus to you.

Diagnosis of Oral Thrush

Your doctor may be able to diagnose oral thrush simply by examining your mouth for the characteristic lesions that it causes.

In some cases, your doctor may take a biopsy of the affected area to confirm the diagnosis. To perform a biopsy, they will scrape off a small portion of the lesion from your mouth. The sample will then be sent to a laboratory to be tested for *C. albicans*.

If your doctor suspects that you have oral thrush in your esophagus, they may use a throat swab culture or endoscopy to confirm the diagnosis.

To perform a throat swab culture, your doctor uses a cotton swab to take a tissue sample from the back of your throat. They then send this sample to a laboratory for testing.

To perform endoscopy, your doctor uses a thin tube with a light and camera attached to it. They insert this "endoscope" through your mouth and into your esophagus to examine it. They may also remove a sample of tissue for analysis.

Treatment for Oral Thrush

To treat oral thrush, your doctor may prescribe one or more of the following medications:

- Fluconazole (Diflucan), an oral antifungal medication.
- Clotrimazole (Mycelex Troche), an antifungal medication that's available as a lozenge.
- Nystatin (Nystop and Nyata), an antifungal mouthwash that you can swish in your mouth or swab in your baby's mouth.
- Itraconazole (Sporanox), an oral antifungal medication that's used to treat people who don't respond to other treatments for oral thrush and people with HIV.
- Amphotericin B (AmBisome and Fungizone), a medication that's used to treat severe cases of oral thrush.

Once you begin treatment, oral thrush usually goes away within a couple of weeks. But in some cases, it can return.

For adults who have recurring cases of oral thrush with no known cause, their healthcare provider will evaluate them for underlying medical conditions that might be contributing to thrush.

Infants may have several episodes of oral thrush in their first year of life.

Home Remedies for Oral Thrush

Your doctor might also recommend home remedies or lifestyle changes to help treat oral thrush or stop it from coming back.

When you're recovering, it's important to practice good oral hygiene. Here are a few tips:

- Brush your teeth with a soft toothbrush to avoid scraping the spots caused by thrush.
- Replace your toothbrush after you finish your treatment for oral thrush, and properly clean your dentures if you wear them, in order to lower your risk of reinfection.
- Avoid mouthwashes or mouth sprays, unless your doctor has prescribed them.

Some home remedies may also help relieve symptoms of thrush in adults.

For example, it might help to rinse your mouth with one of the following:

- Saltwater.
- A solution of water and baking soda.
- A mixture of water and lemon juice.
- A mixture of water and apple cider vinegar.

It might also help to eat yogurt that contains beneficial bacteria or take a probiotic supplement. Talk to a doctor before giving an infant any supplements.

Pictures of Oral Thrush

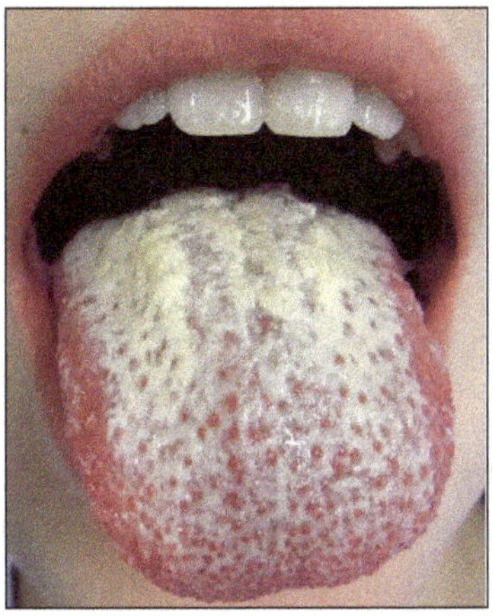

Oral Thrush and Breastfeeding

The same fungus that causes oral thrush can also cause yeast infections on your breasts and nipples.

This fungus can be passed back and forth between mothers and babies during breastfeeding.

If your baby has oral thrush, they can potentially pass the fungus to your breasts or other areas of skin. If you have a breast yeast infection or nipple yeast infection, you can potentially pass the fungus to your baby's mouth or skin.

Also, because yeast can live on the skin without causing an infection, your baby can develop oral thrush without you having any symptoms of a breast or nipple yeast infection.

If you develop a yeast infection on your breasts or nipples, you may experience:

- Pain in your breasts, during and after breastfeeding.
- Itchiness or a burning sensation in or around your nipples.
- White or pale spots on or around your nipples.
- Shiny skin on or around your nipples.
- Flaking skin on or around your nipples.

If your baby develops oral thrush or you develop a breast or nipple yeast infection, it's important to get treatment for both you and your baby. This can help prevent a cycle of transmission.

Your healthcare provider may advise you to do the following:

- Treat your baby with an antifungal medication and apply an antifungal cream, such as terbinafine (Lamisil) or clotrimazole (Lotrimin), to your breasts. Wipe the cream off your breasts before breastfeeding your baby to stop the cream from getting in their mouth.
- Sterilize your baby's pacifiers, teething rings, bottle nipples, and any other items they put in their mouth. If you use a breast pump, sterilize all of its pieces as well.
- Keep your nipples clean and dry between feedings. If you use nursing pads, avoid those that have a plastic liner, which may trap moisture and create favorable conditions for fungus to grow.

Your doctor might also advise you to make lifestyle changes to help treat or prevent oral thrush and other types of yeast infection.

Oral Thrush in Babies

Oral thrush most often affects infants and toddlers. Babies can potentially develop oral thrush after contracting the fungus from their mothers during pregnancy, delivery, or breastfeeding or just from yeast that is naturally present in their environment.

If your baby has oral thrush, they may develop the same signs and symptoms that can affect other people with the condition, including:

- White or yellow spots or patches on their inner cheeks, tongue, tonsils, gums, or lips.
- Slight bleeding if the spots are scraped.
- Soreness or burning in their mouth.
- Dry, cracked skin at the corners of their mouth.

Oral thrush in babies may also cause difficulty feeding and irritability or fussiness.

If you suspect that your baby might have oral thrush, make an appointment with their doctor. If your baby develops oral thrush while you're breastfeeding them, both of you will need antifungal treatments.

Oral Thrush in Adults

Oral thrush is most common in babies and older adults, who tend to have weaker immune systems. But it can occur at any age.

Younger adults can develop oral thrush, especially if they have an impaired immune system. For example, adults are more likely to develop thrush if they have a history of certain medical conditions, medical treatments, or lifestyle habits that weaken their immune system.

In otherwise healthy adults, oral thrush is unlikely to cause serious problems. But if your immune system isn't working well, the infection may spread to other parts of your body.

Risk Factors for Oral Thrush

Babies, toddlers, and older adults are more likely than others to develop oral thrush. Certain medical conditions, medical treatments, and lifestyle factors can also increase your risk of thrush by weakening your immune system or disrupting the balance of microbes in your body.

For example, you may be at heightened risk of thrush if you:

- Have a condition that causes dry mouth.
- Have diabetes, anemia, leukemia, or HIV.
- Take antibiotics, corticosteroids, or immunosuppressant drugs.
- Receive treatments for cancer, such as chemotherapy or radiation therapy.
- Smoke cigarettes.
- Wear dentures.

Complications of Oral Thrush

In people with healthy immune systems, oral thrush rarely causes complications. In severe cases, it may spread to your esophagus.

If your immune system is weakened, you're more likely to develop complications from thrush. Without proper treatment, the fungus that causes thrush may enter your bloodstream and spread to your heart, brain, eyes, or other body parts. This is known as invasive or systemic candidiasis.

Systemic candidiasis can cause problems in the organs it affects. It can also cause a potentially life-threatening condition known as septic shock.

Prevention of Oral Thrush

To reduce your risk of oral thrush, try the following:

- Avoid sharing cups and utensils with others.
- Eat a nutritious diet and practice an overall healthy lifestyle to support the functioning of your immune system.
- Practice good oral hygiene by brushing your teeth twice a day, flossing every day, and visiting your dentist on a regular basis.
- If your mouth is chronically dry, make an appointment with your doctor and follow their recommended treatment plan.
- If you have dentures, remove them before you go to bed, clean them daily, and make sure they fit properly.
- If you have a corticosteroid inhaler, rinse out your mouth or brush your teeth after using it.
- If you have diabetes, take steps to manage your blood sugar levels.

If you develop a yeast infection in another part of your body other than your mouth, get treatment. In some cases, an infection can spread from one part of your body to another.

Oral Thrush and Diet

Some studies suggest that eating certain probiotic foods or taking probiotic supplements might help limit the growth of *C. albicans*. However, more research is needed to learn about the role that probiotics might play in treating or preventing oral thrush.

Some people believe that limiting or avoiding certain foods may also help curb the growth of *C. albicans*. For example, some people have suggested that limiting refined carbohydrates and sugars can help treat or prevent oral thrush and other yeast infections. More research is needed to understand how diet may affect oral thrush.

The "candida diet" has been developed based on these beliefs. However, this diet lacks scientific support.

Vaginal Candidiasis

The vagina is infected by a yeast called *Candida*, usually *Candida albicans*, resulting in a yeast infection called candidiasis.

- Being pregnant or having diabetes or a weakened immune system increases the risk of yeast infections.
- The vagina and vulva may itch, and women often have a thick, white discharge resembling cottage cheese.
- If symptoms suggest a vaginal infection, doctors examine a sample of the discharge and may test it or fluid from the cervix for microorganisms that can cause infection.
- Antifungal drugs—creams, vaginal suppositories, tablets, or capsules—are effective.

Causes of Vaginal Yeast Infection

In women of child-bearing age, yeast infections due to *Candida albicans* are particularly common. This yeast normally resides on the skin or in the intestine. From these areas, it can spread to the vagina. Yeast infections are not transmitted sexually.

Vaginal yeast infections are more likely to occur in women who:

- Are pregnant,
- Have diabetes,
- Have a weakened immune system—suppressed by drugs (such as corticosteroids or chemotherapy drugs) or impaired by a disorder (such as AIDS),
- Use an intrauterine device,
- Wear tight undergarments that do not let air circulate and
- Are taking antibiotics.

Antibiotics taken by mouth tend to kill the bacteria that normally reside in the vagina and that prevent yeast from growing. Thus, using antibiotics increases the risk of developing a yeast infection.

Yeast infections are more likely to occur just before menstrual periods.

After menopause, yeast infections are uncommon except in women who take hormone therapy.

Male sex partners of women with a vaginal yeast infection rarely become infected.

Symptoms of Vaginal Yeast Infection

The vagina and vulva may itch or burn, particularly during sexual intercourse. The genital area may become red and swollen. Women may have a white discharge, often thick and resembling cottage cheese.

Yeast infection symptoms may worsen the week before a menstrual period begins.

Diagnosis of Vaginal Yeast Infection

- A doctor's evaluation.

- Examination of a sample of the discharge and/or fluid from the cervix.

If women have a vaginal discharge that is unusual or that lasts for more than a few days or have other vaginal symptoms, they should see a doctor.

Doctors suspect a yeast infection based on symptoms, such as a thick, white discharge that often resembles cottage cheese. They then ask questions about the discharge, other symptoms, possible causes (such as diabetes, other disorders, and use of antibiotics or hormones), and hygiene.

To confirm the diagnosis, doctors do a pelvic examination. While examining the vagina, the doctor takes a sample of the discharge with a cotton-tipped swab. The sample is examined under a microscope and sometimes cultured (placed in a substance that allows microorganisms to grow). With information from these examinations, the doctor can usually identify the microorganism causing the symptoms.

Usually, the doctor also uses a swab to take a sample of fluid from the cervix (the lower part of the uterus that opens into the vagina). This sample is tested for sexually transmitted infections.

Prevention of Vaginal Yeast Infection

Women who are at high risk of a yeast infection may need to take an antifungal drug by mouth to help prevent yeast infections. Such women include those with the following:

- Diabetes.
- A need to take antibiotics for a long time.
- Repeated yeast infections, particularly in women with a weakened immune system.

Keeping the vulva clean and wearing loose, absorbent cotton clothing that allows air to circulate can reduce moisture, which encourages the growth of yeast, and thus help prevent yeast from growing.

Treatment of Vaginal Yeast Infection

- Antifungal drugs.

Yeast infections are treated with antifungal drugs. They may be used in the following ways:

- Applied as a cream to the affected area.
- Inserted into the vagina as a suppository.
- Taken by mouth.

Butoconazole, clotrimazole, miconazole, and tioconazole are available without a prescription. Oils in these creams and ointments weaken latex-based condoms (but not diaphragms), so women cannot rely on condoms for birth control.

Antifungal drugs (such as fluconazole and itraconazole) taken by mouth require a prescription. A single dose of fluconazole is as effective as the creams and ointments. However, if infections recur often, women may need to take several doses.

Penile Candidiasis

Penile yeast infections can create a range of uncomfortable symptoms, but are often treated quickly by OTC medications, and can be reduced by taking certain steps, such as practicing proper hygiene.

Penile Yeast Infection

A yeast infection is often thought of as a female health problem, but it can affect anyone, including people with a penis.

A penile yeast infection can lead to a wide range of painful and uncomfortable symptoms if not treated. It can also lead to serious complications if the infection spreads to your bloodstream.

Over-the-counter (OTC) medications can often clear up a yeast infection, and some basic prevention steps can help you avoid this fairly common condition.

Symptoms of a Penile Yeast Infection

Some of the most common symptoms of a penile yeast infection include:

- Redness, soreness, or swelling of the penis.
- White, shiny patches at the top of the penis.
- Small red spots at the top of the penis.
- Cracked foreskin.
- Thick, white discharge under the foreskin or other folds of skin.
- Difficulty pulling back the foreskin.
- Itchiness.
- Burning sensation during urination.
- Pain or discomfort during sex.

Redness, itchiness, and pain in the penis can be signs of other more serious conditions, like some sexually transmitted infections (STIs), so do not ignore symptoms once they appear.

An urologist or primary care doctor can diagnose the condition, often in a single appointment.

Causes of Penile Yeast Infection

A yeast infection is usually caused by a fungus called candida. A small amount of candida is usually present in the body. All it takes is an overgrowth of candida to develop a yeast infection.

A moist environment is ideal for candida to spread, according to 2018 research.

Having sex with a person who has a vaginal yeast infection without using a condom can also cause a penile yeast infection. However, you can also develop an infection without sexual activity.

Risk Factors for a Penile Yeast Infection

Aside from sex with a partner who has a yeast infection, several other risk factors can increase your odds of developing a penile yeast infection, such as:

- Not cleaning your genitals or bathing regularly.
- Having a weakened immune function due to certain medications or health conditions.
- Using antibiotics long term.
- Wearing wet clothing or tight-fitting underwear.
- Using skin products or soaps that cause skin irritation.
- Having diabetes.
- Using lubricated condoms.
- Being uncircumcised.
- Having obesity.

Diagnosis of a Penile Yeast Infection

Once you make an appointment, a doctor will ask you about your symptoms and likely examine your genitals. Some of the white substance that forms on the penis may be examined under a microscope to confirm the type of fungus causing the symptoms, according to 2022 research.

If you cannot get in to see a doctor or a urologist, consider a visit to an urgent care center or the emergency room. The earlier the problem is diagnosed and treatment begins, the more likely it is you can avoid complications.

It's not recommended for a person to diagnose themselves and start treatment on their own. If symptoms of a yeast infection are present, contact a doctor. If symptoms are allowed to persist, complications can become very uncomfortable.

Treat of Penile Yeast Infection

In most cases, topical antifungal ointments and creams are enough to clear up an infection. Some of the antifungal creams recommended for a yeast infection include:

- Miconazole (Lotrimin AF, Cruex, Desenex, Ting Antifungal).
- Imidazole (Canesten, Selezen).
- Clotrimazole (Lotrimin AF, Anti-Fungal, Cruex, Desenex, Lotrimin AF Ringworm).

Most of these are available as OTC medications, which mean you will not need a prescription. More serious or long-term infections may require prescription-strength medication.

Oral fluconazole (Diflucan) and hydrocortisone cream may be advised in serious infections, like those that have developed into a potentially serious condition called balanitis.

Most antifungal creams are well tolerated and unlikely to cause any serious side effects. Check the label, however, and ask a doctor and pharmacist what to look out for in case you have a bad reaction.

Recurrent Yeast Infections

Yeast infections sometimes return after they seem to have been cured. If this happens, your doctor will likely recommend a few weeks of daily treatments followed by a few months of weekly treatments.

In some cases, treatment for recurrent yeast infections can last up to 6 months.

If your infection does not respond well to an antifungal ointment and you are uncircumcised, you may be advised to have an adult male circumcision, according to 2016 research. Though this surgical procedure is usually done on infants, it can be done safely on people of any age.

Diabetes and Yeast Infections

Factors like diabetes and a suppressed immune system may contribute to your yeast infection risk, according to 2019 research.

If you have diabetes, work with a healthcare professional to make sure your blood sugar levels are well-managed. If you have a suppressed immune system, a doctor can recommend ways to help keep your immune system as healthy as possible.

Complications of a Penile Yeast Infection

If left untreated, a penile yeast infection can lead to some serious complications.

Balanitis

One of the potential complications of a penile yeast infection is balanitis. Balanitis is an inflammation of the foreskin or head of the penis. Diabetes can increase your risk for balanitis.

If balanitis is not treated effectively, scarring of the foreskin can occur. It can also cause adhesions on the penis.

Balanitis can be painful and make urinating more difficult. If untreated, it can cause swollen and painful glands as well as weakness and fatigue.

Invasive Candidiasis

A yeast infection may enter the bloodstream. This is known as candidemia or invasive candidiasis.

This is most common in people who wait to receive treatment until the infection has spread beyond the penis. It is also more common in those with weakened immune systems.

If you've been in a hospital and used a catheter to urinate, you may be more likely to face invasive candidiasis. This advanced form of yeast infection is very serious.

Oral antifungal medications may be needed for several weeks. In some cases, the drugs are administered intravenously.

Persistence of Penile Yeast Infection Last

If your infection is treated early and responds well to antifungal medication, it can clear up within 7 to 14 days.

If you are sexually active, your partner should also be treated for a yeast infection to avoid passing the infection on to them, or back to you.

If you get repeated yeast infections and can rule out causes like hygiene and sexual contact, talk with a doctor about other possible causes. You may have an underlying health condition, such as diabetes.

Prevention of a Penile Yeast Infection

You can help prevent a penile yeast infection by avoiding sexual contact with a partner who has a yeast infection.

You should also avoid having sex with anyone while you have an active yeast infection, as you could pass the infection back to your partner. This could cause the two of you to pass an infection back and forth.

To lower the risk of getting a yeast infection or passing one along, do the following:

- Wear an external condom each time you have sex to help reduce your chances of developing a yeast infection.
- Practice good hygiene, and keep your penis and genitals clean and dry.
- If you are uncircumcised, clean under the foreskin with soap and water, and return your foreskin to its usual position after you have sexual intercourse.

Cutaneous Candidiasis

Different types of bacteria and fungi live and grow on your skin. Most of them aren't dangerous. Your body requires the majority of them to carry out normal functions. However, some can cause infections when they begin to multiply uncontrollably.

The *Candida* fungus is one of these potentially harmful organisms. When an overgrowth of *Candida* develops on the skin, an infection can occur. This condition is known as candidiasis of the skin, or cutaneous candidiasis.

Candidiasis of the skin often causes a red, itchy rash to form, most commonly in the folds of the skin. This rash may also spread to other areas of the body. While the symptoms are often bothersome, they can usually be treated with improved hygiene and antifungal creams or powders.

Symptoms of Candidiasis of the Skin

The main symptom of candidiasis of the skin is a rash. The rash often causes redness and intense itching. In some cases, the infection can cause the skin to become cracked and sore. Blisters and pustules may also occur.

The rash can affect various parts the body, but it's most likely to develop in the folds of the skin. This includes areas in the armpits, in the groin, between the fingers, and under the breasts. *Candida* can also cause infections in the nails, edges of the nails, and corners of the mouth.

Other conditions that may resemble candidiasis of the skin include:

- Ringworm.
- Hives.
- Herpes.
- Diabetes-Related Skin Conditions.
- Contact Dermatitis.
- Seborrheic Dermatitis.
- Eczema.
- Psoriasis.

Causes of Candidiasis of the Skin

Candidiasis of the skin develops when the skin becomes infected with *Candida*. A small amount of *Candida* fungi naturally live on the skin. When this type of fungus begins to multiply uncontrollably, however, it can cause an infection. This may occur because of:

- Warm weather.
- Tight clothing.
- Poor hygiene.
- Infrequent undergarment changes.
- Obesity.
- The use of antibiotics that kill harmless bacteria that keeps candida under control.
- The use of corticosteroids or other medications that affect the immune system.
- A weakened immune system as a result of diabetes, pregnancy, or another medical condition.

- Incomplete drying of damp or wet skin.

Candida fungi thrive and grow in warm, moist areas. This is why the condition often affects areas where there are folds of skin.

Babies can also develop candidiasis of the skin, especially on the buttocks. A diaper tends to provide an ideal environment for *Candida*.

Candidiasis of the skin usually isn't contagious. However, people with weakened immune systems may develop the condition after touching the skin of an infected person. Those with compromised immune systems are also more likely to develop a severe infection as a result of candidiasis.

Diagnosis Candidiasis of the Skin

Your doctor will likely be able to make a diagnosis simply by performing a physical examination. During the exam, they'll inspect the location of your rash and the appearance of your skin.

Your doctor may also want to perform a skin culture before making a diagnosis of candidiasis of the skin. During a skin culture, your doctor will rub a cotton swab over the affected area and collect a skin sample. The sample will then be sent to a laboratory to be tested for the presence of *Candida*.

Treatment of Candidiasis of the Skin

Candidiasis of the skin can usually be prevented with home remedies, the most important of which is proper hygiene. Washing the skin regularly and drying the skin thoroughly can prevent the skin from becoming too moist. This is vital to keeping *Candida* infections at bay.

There are many lifestyle changes you can make to both prevent and treat a candidiasis infection:

- Quickly change out of damp clothing, such as swimsuits or sweaty workout clothes.
- Change your socks and undergarments regularly.
- Wear loose-fitting clothing.
- Use gentle and scent-free soap on affected areas.
- Add probiotics to your diet.
- Reduce the amount of sugar in your diet.

Since abnormal blood sugar levels can contribute to the development of Candida infections, keeping your blood sugar under control may also help relieve symptoms. You may be able to lower your blood sugar by reducing the amount of sugar in your diet and by exercising for 30 minutes at least three times per week. If you have diabetes, it's important to continue following your doctor's instructions as you may need to start receiving oral medications or an increased amount of insulin.

In severe or persistent cases of candidiasis, your doctor may recommend using an antifungal cream or powder that can be applied to your skin. Over-the-counter antifungal creams that are often recommended include clotrimazole (Mycelex), miconazole (Monistat), and tioconazole (Vagistat). This type of treatment can kill Candida and reduce the spread of the infection.

Your doctor may prescribe an antifungal cream such as nystatin or ketoconazole if the over-the-counter treatments aren't effective. If the infection has already spread to areas inside your body, such as your throat or mouth, you may need to take an oral antifungal to get rid of it.

Cutaneous Candidiasis in Babies

Cutaneous candidiasis (or candidiasis present on skin, nails, or hair) is a common occurrence in infants and babies.

Candidiasis-related diaper rash is one of the most frequently occurring candidiasis infections in babies. This rash is typically red with a well-defined border, and normally lasts more than three days. Treatment includes changing the infant's diaper frequently and allowing them to wear loose-fitting clothes on top of the diaper. The antifungal nystatin may be prescribed.

Oral thrush is another common occurrence in newborns and infants under 6 months old. Symptoms can include cracked skin in the corners of the mouth and whitish patches on the lips, tongue, or inside of the cheeks. Your doctor can prescribe an antifungal medication that's applied to the infant's mouth several times a day.

If candidiasis infection is left untreated, it can enter the bloodstream and spread. See your doctor if you believe your baby has candidiasis.

Cutaneous Candidiasis in Children

Although healthy children have strong immune systems, a 2010 study found that the rate of topical fungal infections among children is increasing rapidly. Children sometimes develop candidiasis infections after receiving antibiotics that treat another condition. Children who suck their thumbs may be prone to developing candidiasis infections in or around their nail beds.

If your child is 9 months or older and has reoccurring thrush or skin infections, this could point to an underlying health concern, such as HIV or another problem with the immune system. Older children with frequent or severe skin infections should also be tested for diabetes.

Candida Nail Infection

A fungal nail infection is a common condition that can leave you with brittle, discolored nails, usually on your toes.

Its formal name is onychomycosis, and it's a lot like athlete's foot. But instead of affecting the skin on the bottom of your feet or between your toes, it invades your nails.

Fungi are tiny organisms you can only see through a microscope. Many different types can cause a nail infection. Sometimes they live on your skin and don't make any trouble. But if you have a lot in one area, you might get infected.

Don't be embarrassed if you have toenail or fingernail fungus. It's way more common than you think.

Types of Fungal Nail Infections

There are four main kinds of fungal nail infection. Each looks slightly different:

- Distal or lateral subungual onychomycosis: This is the most common kind. It results from a fungus called a dermatophyte. You can get it in your fingernails or toenails. It starts in the nail bed, underneath the nail. You'll see a yellowish colored area that spreads from the edges of the nail to the center, and places where it comes apart from the nail bed.
- White superficial onychomycosis: This is less common and only affects the nail surface, mainly on your toenails. It starts as white spots, which become powdery and cause the nail to crumble.
- Proximal subungual onychomycosis: This appears first as white spots in the center of the nail bed at the cuticle. They move outward as the finger or toenail grows. It's rare and usually affects people who have immune system problems, like HIV infection.
- Candidal onychomycosis: Yeast causes this infection that usually affects your fingernails. The area around the nails is often swollen and inflamed, and the nails may come off entirely. It tends to happen to nails that have been damaged by an injury or another infection.

Fungal Nail Infection Symptoms

Symptoms are different depending on which type of fungal nail infection you have. They usually start mild and get more serious.

- At first, you may only see a white or yellow spot under your nail. Over time, this spreads and can turn your whole nail white, yellow, green, or black.
- The nail may thicken and could be hard to trim.
- It may start to curl up or down or loosen from the nail bed.
- Your nail could become brittle and crumble when you touch it.
- Your nail may become misshapen.
- You may notice a bad smell.

It's easy to ignore fungal nail infections at first, since you may not have any pain. But if you don't treat them, it can hurt to put any pressure on the area. If an infection gets bad enough, it could even become hard to walk.

Fungal Nail Infection Causes

It's a good idea to wash your hands and feet often. Use soap, and make sure you get between your fingers and toes.

Keep your fingernails and toenails short and trimmed straight across.

Wear socks that wick away (absorb) moisture. If your feet sweat a lot, change your socks once or twice a day, or take off your shoes and let your feet cool when you have the chance.

Use antifungal powder or spray on your feet as well as in your shoes. Throw away old pairs of closed-toe shoes since fungi might be living in them.

If you get manicures at nail salons, visit only the ones that disinfect tools after each client. You can also bring your own file and clippers from home. Ask that your cuticles not be cut, since this can cause tiny breaks in the skin that let germs in.

Don't share towels if someone else in your family has nail fungus. This will pass around the infection.

See your doctor if you think you have nail fungus. You may need a prescription to treat it, whether that means taking a medicine by mouth or using a special cream. In severe cases, your nail may need to be removed so a healthy new one can grow in its place. Doctors can also use lasers to treat nail fungus.

You get an infection when a crack in your nail or the skin around it allows fungus to get inside and grow.

Since fungus thrives in dark, warm places, your toenails are more likely to be affected than your fingernails. Your toes also have less blood flow than your fingers, which makes it harder for your body to pick up on and prevent an infection.

You're more likely to get a fungal nail infection if you:

- Are a man.
- Are older. Nails become more brittle and likely to crack as you age.
- Have a weak immune system or ongoing health problems like diabetes.
- Wear shoes that make your feet hot and sweaty.
- Walk barefoot through gym showers, swimming pools, and locker rooms. These are places where fungus spreads easily.
- Live with someone who has a fungal infection.
- Have athlete's foot. The fungus that causes it can spread to your nails.
- Recently had an injury or surgery on your nail, or had a previous infection.
- Wear plastic gloves or keep your hands wet for long periods of time.

Fungal Nail Infection Treatment

See your doctor if you think you have nail fungus. It can be tough to get rid of, and you're more likely to have success with a prescription. Treatments include:

- Oral antifungals: The doctor may give you a pill to kill fungus in your whole body. This is usually the best way to get rid of a nail infection. Treatment may last 2 months for an infection in your fingernails, or 3 months if it's in your toenails.

- Topical antifungals: You rub or brush these medicines onto your nails. They may work for a mild infection, but they can't get deep enough into the nail to cure a more serious one. You might use a topical treatment in combination with a pill.
- Surgery: If other treatments don't work, the doctor may need to remove your nail entirely and let a healthy one grow back in its place. The new nail could also get infected.
- Laser or photodynamic therapy: Doctors are studying newer treatments that use special light to try to kill the fungus.

Fungal Nail Infection Prevention

It's a good idea to wash your hands and feet often. Use soap, and make sure you get between your fingers and toes.

Keep your fingernails and toenails short and trimmed straight across.

Wear socks that wick away moisture. If your feet sweat a lot, change your socks once or twice a day, or take off your shoes and let your feet cool when you have the chance.

Use antifungal powder or spray on your feet as well as in your shoes. Throw away old pairs of closed-toe shoes since fungi might be living in them.

If you get manicures at nail salons, visit only the ones that disinfect tools after each client. You can also bring your own file and clippers from home. Ask them not to cut your cuticles, since this can cause tiny breaks in the skin that let germs in.

Don't share towels if someone else in your family has nail fungus. This will pass around the infection.

Fungal Nail Infection Complications

It can take a year or more for your nails to look like they did before the infection. And you may continue to have problems:

- The fungus can come back.
- Your nails may be permanently discolored or misshapen.
- The infection may spread to other parts of your body.

It's especially important to take care of a fungal nail infection if you have diabetes. You're at greater risk of getting a serious skin infection.

Chronic Mucocutaneous Candidiasis

Chronic mucocutaneous candidiasis is persistent or recurrent candidal infection due to inherited T-cell defects. Autoimmune and endocrine disorders may develop in its recessive form. Diagnosis is based on recurrent, unexplained candida infections. Treatment includes antifungal drugs and treatment of any endocrine and autoimmune disorders.

Chronic mucocutaneous candidiasis is a primary immunodeficiency disorder that involves T cell defects. Some patients also have deficient humoral immunity (sometimes called antibody deficiency), characterized by abnormal antibody responses to polysaccharide antigens despite normal immunoglobulin levels.

Inheritance may be:

- Autosomal dominant: Involving a mutation in the signal transducer and activator of transcription 1 gene (STAT1).
- Autosomal recessive: Involving a mutation in the autoimmune regulator gene (AIRE).

In the **recessive form** (autoimmune polyendocrinopathy–candidosis-ectodermal dystrophy), autoimmune manifestations typically develop; they include endocrine disorders (eg, hypoparathyroidism, adrenal insufficiency, hypogonadism, thyroid disorders, diabetes), alopecia areata, pernicious anemia, and hepatitis. Mutations may also occur in genes that encode various proteins involved in the innate immune response to fungi—notably, the following:

- PTPN22 (protein tyrosine phosphatase, non-receptor type 22 [also called LYP, or lymphoid tyrosine phosphatase], which is involved in T-cell–receptor signalling).
- Dectin-1 (an innate pattern recognition receptor essential for the control of fungal infections).
- CARD9 (caspase recruitment domain-containing protein 9, which is an adaptor molecule important in the production of interleukin (IL)-17 and for protection against fungal invasion).

Patients (dominant and recessive) have cutaneous anergy to *Candida*, absent proliferative responses to *Candida* antigen (but normal proliferative responses to mitogens), and intact antibody response to *Candida* and other antigens. Mucocutaneous candidiasis recurs or persists, usually beginning during infancy but sometimes during early adulthood. Life span is not affected.

Symptoms and Signs of Chronic Mucocutaneous Candidiasis

Thrush is common, as are candidal infections of the scalp, skin, nails, and gastrointestinal and vaginal mucosa. Severity varies. Nails may be thickened, cracked, and discolored, with edema and erythema of the surrounding periungual tissue, resembling clubbing. Skin lesions are crusted, pustular, erythematous, and hyperkeratotic. Scalp lesions may result in scarring alopecia.

Infants often present with refractory thrush, candidal diaper rash, or both.

Candidal Infections

Candidiasis (Nail Infection)

Candidal nail infections can involve the full thickness of the nail plate (onychomycosis), the edges of the nail (paronychia), or both.

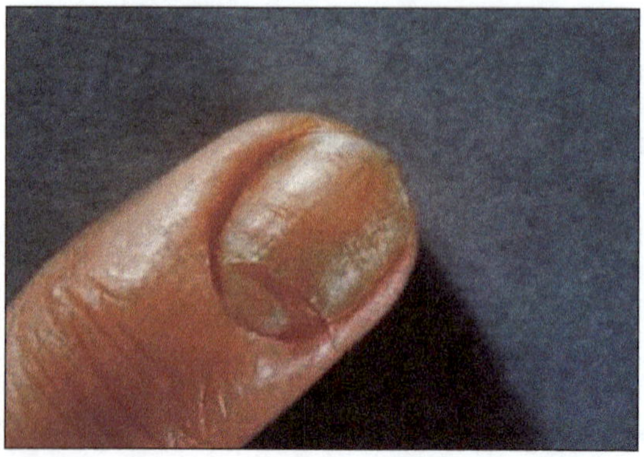

Thrush

Creamy white patches are seen inside the mouth and may bleed when scraped off. This finding is typical of thrush, which is caused by infection with Candida.

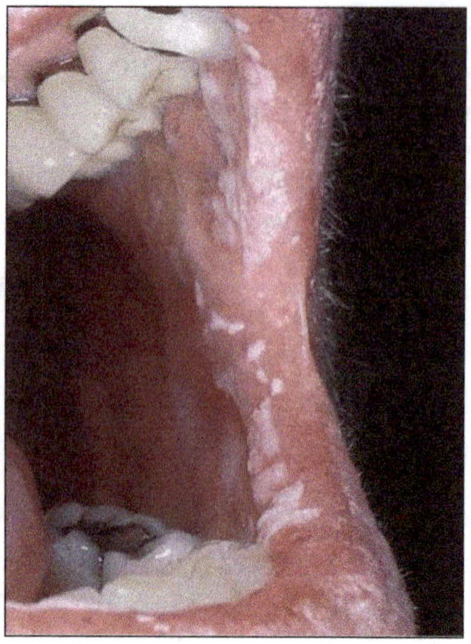

Candida Esophagitis

Diffuse whitish plaques are typical of Candida esophagitis.

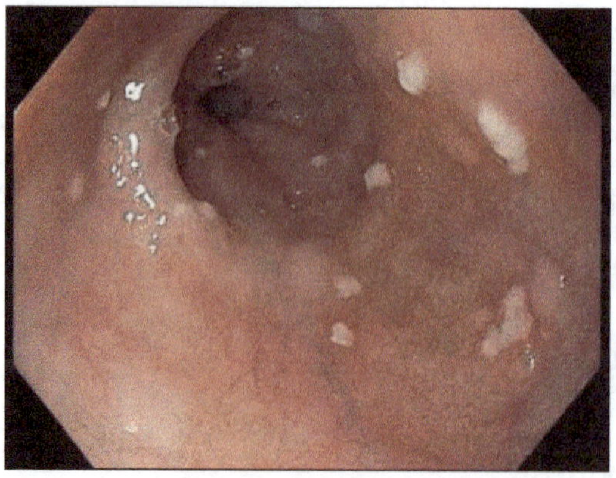

Diagnosis of Chronic Mucocutaneous Candidiasis

Clinical Evaluation

Candidal lesions are confirmed by standard tests (eg, potassium hydroxide wet mount of scrapings).

Diagnosis of chronic mucocutaneous candidiasis is based on the presence of recurrent candidal skin or mucosal lesions when no other known causes of candidal infection (eg, diabetes, antibiotic use) are present.

Patients are screened for endocrine disorders based on clinical suspicion.

Genetic testing is done if clinical suspicion is high and other common causes of the patient's clinical symptoms have been eliminated. If an *AIRE* mutation is detected, screening can be offered to the patient's siblings and children.

Treatment of Chronic Mucocutaneous Candidiasis

- Antifungal drugs and
- Treatment of endocrine and autoimmune manifestations.

Usually, the infections of chronic mucocutaneous candidiasis can be controlled with a topical antifungal, if patients have a poor response to topical antifungals, long-term treatment with a systemic antifungal drug (eg, amphotericin B, fluconazole, ketoconazole) may be needed. Immune globulin should be considered if patients have antibody deficiency.

Autoimmune (including endocrine) manifestations are treated aggressively.

Hematopoietic stem cell transplantation has rarely been successful and could be considered as last-line treatment in severe cases.

- Inheritance of chronic mucocutaneous candidiasis is autosomal dominant or recessive.
- Patients with the recessive form can have autoimmune (including endocrine) manifestations.
- Diagnose the disorder by confirming mucocutaneous candidiasis and excluding other causes.
- Treat candidiasis with antifungal drugs (using a systemic drug if needed), and treat autoimmune manifestations.

Malassezia Folliculitis

Malassezia folliculitis, also known as pityrosporum folliculitis, is an infection of the pilosebaceous unit caused by lipophilic Malassezia yeasts particularly *M. globosa, M. sympodialis* and *M. restricta*. Malassezia yeast is normal inhabitants of the human skin surface and only cause disease under specific conditions.

Malassezia yeasts have been linked to a number of other skin diseases including seborrhoeic dermatitis and pityriasis versicolor.

Malassezia Folliculitis

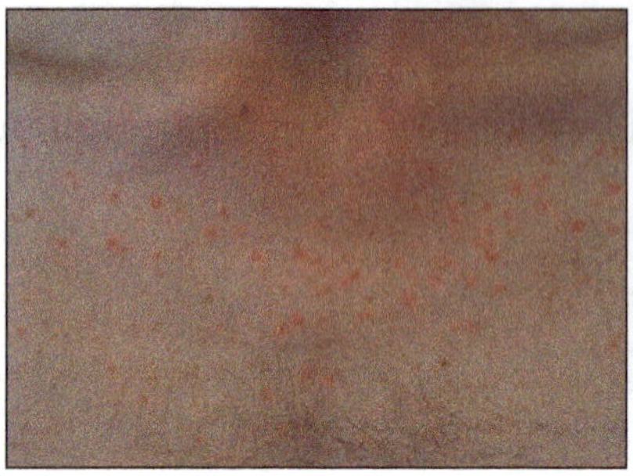

(a) Malassezia folliculitis

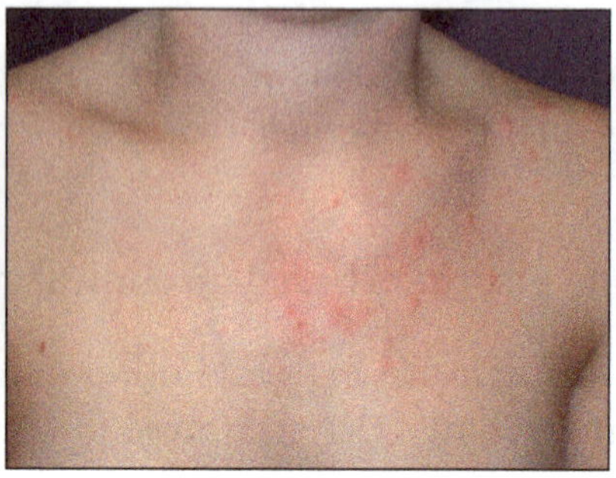

(b) Malassezia folliculitis

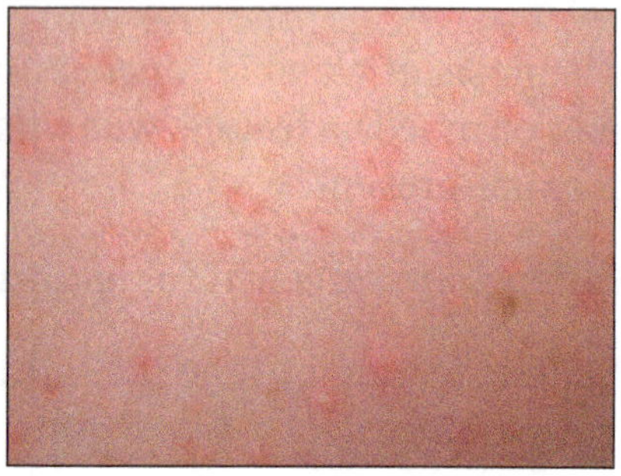

(c) Malassezia folliculitis

Risk Factors of Malassezia Folliculitis

Malassezia folliculitis is most commonly seen in adolescent and young adult males.

Risk factors for developing *Malassezia* folliculitis include:

- Hot humid climate.
- High sebum production.
- Hyperhidrosis (excessive sweating).
- Occlusion from emollients and sunscreens.
- Antibiotic use.
- Immunosuppression including topical and oral steroid use and HIV.

Clinical Features of Malassezia Folliculitis

Malassezia folliculitis presents as small, uniform, itchy papules and pustules particularly on the upper back and chest. Other sites involved can include the forehead/hair line, chin, neck, and extensor aspect of the upper limbs. This is a monomorphic eruption and comedones are not seen, distinguishing this condition from acne vulgaris.

Wood lamp examination may demonstrate a yellow-green fluorescence.

Dermoscopy features have been described and include:

- Papules and pustules based on hair follicles.
- Perifollicular erythema.
- Perilesional scale.
- Hypopigmented and coiled/looped hairs.

Diagnosis of Malassezia Folliculitis

Clinical examination raises the diagnosis. Laboratory investigations on skin scraping, tape stripping, swab, or skin biopsy confirm the presence of yeasts as bacterial folliculitis and steroid acne can be clinically similar.

- Potassium hydroxide preparation of skin scrapings may reveal budding yeasts. Hyphae are rarely seen.
- Other stains such as the May-Grünwald-Giema stain are less commonly used.
- Culture of Malassezia species typically requires special media for growth, so is not routinely performed.
- Yeast are seen within the hair follicle and possibly the surrounding dermis on histopathological examination

Differential Diagnosis of Malassezia Folliculitis

Diagnosis of *Malassezia* folliculitis is often delayed due to its clinical resemblance to:

- Acne vulgaris.
- Steroid acne.
- Bacterial folliculitis.

Treatment of Malassezia Folliculitis

It is important to address any predisposing factors at the outset, as *Malassezia* folliculitis has a tendency to recur.

Topical treatments such as selenium sulfide shampoo, econazole solution and topical ketoconazole are effective in the majority of cases but may require a longer course than systemic agents. Ongoing weekly application may be particularly useful as maintenance therapy to prevent recurrence.

Oral treatment may be more effective than topical, although results of clinical trials have not consistently shown this. Fluconazole is used more commonly than itraconazole due to its superior side effect profile.

Isotretinoin and photodynamic therapy (PDT) have been used with some success in small case series of recalcitrant disease.

Prevention of Malassezia folliculitis

Recurrence is common, even after successful treatment.

Long-term prophylaxis with topical agents may be considered in those at high-risk or with multiple recurrences.

Periodic re-evaluation of predisposing factors is recommended.

Seborrhoeic Dermatitis

Seborrheic (seb-o-REE-ik) dermatitis is a common skin condition that mainly affects your scalp. It causes scaly patches, inflamed skin and stubborn dandruff. It usually affects oily areas of the body, such as the face, sides of the nose, eyebrows, ears, eyelids and chest. This condition can be irritating but it's not contagious, and it doesn't cause permanent hair loss.

Seborrheic dermatitis may go away without treatment. Or you may need to use medicated shampoo or other products long term to clear up symptoms and prevent flare-ups.

Seborrheic dermatitis is also called dandruff, seborrheic eczema and seborrheic psoriasis. When it occurs in infants, it's called cradle cap.

Seborrheic Dermatitis on the Face

Seborrheic dermatitis causes a rash of oily patches with yellow or white scales. The rash may look darker or lighter in people with brown or Black skin and redder in those with white skin.

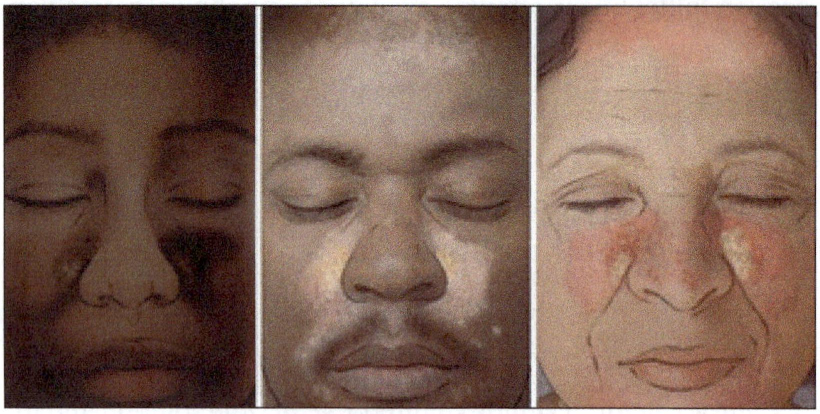

Seborrheic dermatitis on the face.

Symptoms

Seborrheic dermatitis signs and symptoms may include:

- Flaking skin (dandruff) on your scalp, hair, eyebrows, beard or mustache.
- Patches of greasy skin covered with flaky white or yellow scales or crust on the scalp, face, sides of the nose, eyebrows, ears, eyelids, chest, armpits, groin area or under the breasts.
- Rash that may look darker or lighter in people with brown or Black skin and redder in those with white skin.
- Ring-shaped (annular) rash, for a type called petaloid seborrheic dermatitis.
- Itchiness (pruritus).

The signs and symptoms of seborrheic dermatitis tend to flare with stress, fatigue or a change of season.

Doctor Consultation

See your health care provider if:

- You're so uncomfortable that you're losing sleep or are distracted from your daily routines.
- Your condition makes you feel embarrassed or anxious.
- You think your skin is infected.
- You've tried self-care steps, but your symptoms persist.

Causes

The exact cause of seborrheic dermatitis isn't clear. It may be due to the yeast Malassezia, excess oil in the skin or a problem in the immune system.

Risk Factors

Risk factors for seborrheic dermatitis include:

- Stress.
- Fatigue.
- A change of season.
- Nervous system conditions, such as Parkinson's disease.
- Having a mental health condition, such as depression.
- Immune system disorders, such as HIV infection.
- Recovery from stressful medical conditions, such as a heart attack.

White Piedra

White piedra is an uncommon yeast infection of the hair. Several species of a fungus that live in soil or dirty water can cause white piedra.

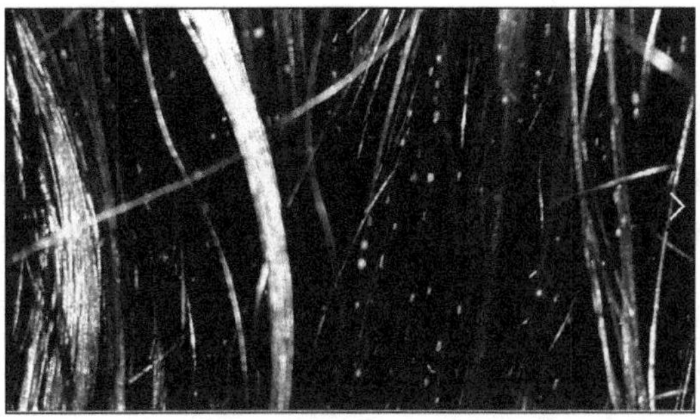

Piedra is the Spanish word for stone. White piedra appears as white or light brown stones that loosely attach to the tip of a hair shaft and may group to form clusters. The stones, which people sometimes call concretions or nodules, feel gritty and are easy to remove.

White piedra occurs more often in warm and tropical regions of the world, such as South America, Africa, and the southeastern United States. The infection can affect people of all ages, genders, and ethnicities.

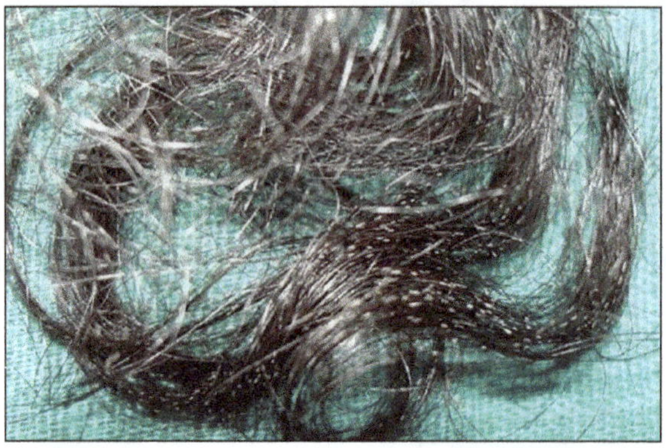

Although white piedra is a relatively harmless condition, without treatment, it can lead to brittle and damaged hair. People can treat it by shaving the affected area and applying an antifungal medication.

In this article, we provide images of white piedra. We also examine the symptoms, causes, and treatment of the condition.

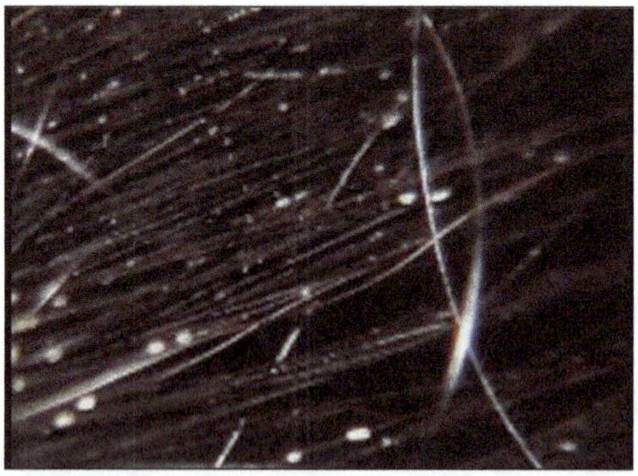

Symptoms

The main symptom of white piedra is the formation of clusters of tiny nodules along the hair shafts.

These rock-like structures appear white, gray, or tan. The stones are soft, feel gritty to the touch, and are easy to remove. However, removal may cause the affected hair shafts to split or break.

White piedra may develop on any area of hair on the body, such as:

- Scalp hair.
- Eyebrows and eyelashes.

- Beard.
- Mustache.
- Underarm hair.
- Pubic hair.

Difference from Similar Conditions

It is easy to confuse white piedra with other skin and hair conditions. However, there are some key differences between them.

- Head and body lice and their shell casings — known as nits — may resemble white piedra stones. However, nits are not as easy to remove as white piedra stones, and lice cause severe itching while white piedra does not. Also, with a lice infection, small white bugs that resemble crabs may be visible to the naked eye.
- Ringworm is a fungal infection of the scalp that appears as a scaly, itchy, ring shaped bald patch.
- Trichomycosis is the colonization of bacteria in the sweat glands. It causes yellow or red concretions with a rancid odor.
- Monilethrix is a rare genetic hair shaft defect that gives the hair a beaded appearance and results in patches of hair loss.
- Dandruff_causes a dry, flaky, itchy scalp. White flakes often fall from the scalp onto a person's face and clothing. Conversely, white piedra remains in the affected area.
- Black piedra is similar to white piedra, but the stones on the hair shafts are brown-black and challenging to remove. Black piedra mainly affects the hair on the scalp, whereas white piedra can affect all areas of hair on the body.
- Hair casts are white, narrow, and cylinder-shaped structures. While hair casts encircle the hair shaft, white piedra does not. Hair casts slide easily along the hair shaft and do not result in hair breakage or damage.

Causes

A species of fungus called *Trichosporon* causes white piedra. *Trichosporon* fungi occur widely in nature, particularly in soil, lake water, and plants. The fungus can also be present in:

- Air.
- Rivers or stagnant water.
- Vegetation.
- Human and animal skin or stool.
- Sewage.

Transmission

White piedra can spread to people when they come into contact with contaminated:

- Water
- Soil
- Plants
- Animals

The spread of white piedra directly from person to person is uncommon. However, it is possible to transmit the infection in the genital region through sexual activity.

After a person is exposed, the fungus needs the right conditions to survive and colonize human hair.

Practices that can lead to colonization and result in white piedra infection include:

- Infrequent bathing or poor personal hygiene.
- Bathing in stagnant water.
- Frequent use of oil applications to the hair.
- Irregular combing habits or matted hair.
- Covering wet hair with a veil or turban.

Risk Factors

White piedra is more common in temperate and semitropical climates. These areas include:

- South America
- Africa
- Europe
- Middle East
- Southeast Asia
- India
- Japan
- Southeastern United States

Additional risk factors for getting a white piedra infection include:

- Inability to wash or bathe frequently.

- Working in unsanitary conditions.
- Excessive sweating.
- Poor personal hygiene.
- Long hair.

Most reports of white piedra have been in children and young adults, particularly females who regularly wear headbands. Also, women who immediately tie and cover wet hair and their scalp with a veil have a higher chance of developing white piedra.

Diagnosis

Individuals who suspect that they have white piedra should see a doctor.

A doctor can diagnose white piedra by conducting a physical examination. They may also recommend microscopic testing of the affected hair to confirm a diagnosis.

Treatment

Shaving the affected area is the preferred treatment for white piedra. Medicated shampoos and lotions may be effective when shaving is not an option for cosmetic, personal, or cultural reasons.

A person can treat white piedra with antifungal lotions and creams. Options may include:

- Clotrimazole 1%.
- Miconazole 2%.
- Ketoconazole 2% shampoo or lotion.
- Ciclopirox.
- Selenium sulfide 2%.

Topical medications do not work for some individuals. A doctor may prescribe an oral antifungal medication, such as itraconazole or terbinafine, to treat persistent white piedra infections.

White piedra of the genitals often recurs, so combining shaving with a short course of a topical antifungal is often necessary for a complete cure.

The fungus may remain in clothing and bedding. A person should throw infected underwear away and disinfect other garments, linen, and towels to help prevent reinfection.

Home Remedies

There are no effective home remedies for treating white piedra. This type of hair infection requires medical evaluation and antifungal medication.

Prevention

White piedra infections will often come back, especially when they can pass between family members. Reinfection is usually the result of sharing combs, hair products or accessories, pillows, and linens.

Several measures can help prevent a person from both initial infection and reinfection with white piedra. These measures include:

- Avoiding sharing brushes, combs, and other hair accessories.
- Wearing loose cotton underwear and changing twice if prone to excessive perspiration during the summer months or in humid conditions.
- Using aluminum chloride hexahydrate (Drysol) to help minimize excessive sweating.
- Drying the skin and hair thoroughly after bathing.
- Drying the scalp hair completely before tying, wrapping, or covering the hair.
- Cleaning all clothing, bedding, and towels that come into contact with the affected areas of hair.

Black Piedra

Piedraia hortae is a superficial fungus that exists in the soils of tropical and subtropical environments and affects both sexes of all ages. The fungus grows very slowly, forming dark hyphae, which contain chlamydoconidia cells and black colonies when grown on agar. Piedraia hortae is a dermatophyte and causes a superficial fungal infection known as black piedra, which causes the formation of black nodules on the hair shaft and leads to progressive weakening of the hair. The infection usually infects hairs on the scalp and beard, but other varieties tend to grow on pubic hairs. The infection is usually treated with cutting or shaving of the hair and followed by the application of anti-fungal and topical agents. The fungus is used for cosmetic purposes to darken hair in some societies as a symbol of attractiveness.

Morphology

When grown on agar at 25 °C (77 °F) *Piedraia hortae* grows very slowly to form black-greenish, limited and pointed colonies. *Piedraia hortae* taken from infected hairs have dark brown nodules, which are made up of ascostroma. The nodules have a gritty feel, organized in a stromatic fashion and have a high concentration of chitin and melanoid pigments. The colonies produce a red pigment and remain smooth and covered with short aerial hyphae. Microscopically, *P. hortae* produces short, dark hyphae containing thick-walled resting cells. The ascomata consist of irregularly shaped pseudothecia that are black in colour. Each ascoma contains a single ascus containing eight ascospores. The ascospores are dark, curved and become very narrow at the ends forming whip-like appendages. Affected hairs develop stone-like black nodules affixed to the hair shaft that cause weakness of the hair. Infected hairs treated with potassium hydroxide fluoresce under ultraviolet light despite that the fungus itself does not normally fluoresce. Fluorescence of the piedra indicates secondary contamination by bacteria. Identification is easily achieved by microscopic examination of the hair nodules, and can be confirmed by sequence analysis of the nuclear ribosomal internal transcribed spacer region.

Pathology

Piedraia hortae causes the formation of nodules on the hair shaft, a clinical superficial disease commonly known as black piedra. Black piedra is usually seen in tropical regions and it usually targets humans of all ages and targets the scalp, moustache and occasionally pubic hair. The source of the infection is usually in soils, poor hygiene, long hair, cultural use of veils and the application of plant oils to wet hair favours the growth of the infection. Black piedra is a superficial fungal infection, which means that it is restricted to the stratum corneum and causes no inflammation. The infection of the hair shaft results in the formation of nodules on the scalp, moustache and pubic hair. The nodules are hard and gritty, which produce a metallic sound when the hair is combed. The nodules colonize the hair shaft, which causes progressive weakness of the hair and leads to breakage of the hair in severe cases, which can lead to hair loss and baldness. The fungus also has the potential to destroy the cuticular layers of the hair and move into the cortex. *Piedraia hortae* survives in the scalp is due to the slow rate of the keratin degradation near the cortex and the compact formation of the nodules and the hyphae are tightly packed in black piedra cases. The initial invasion of human hair by *P. hortae* is achieved by using eroding hyphae, which force their way beneath or between the cuticular layer. The force applied between or beneath the hair cuticle arises from the growth of the fungus itself. The breakdown of keratin is mainly due to enzymatic processes and corresponds to the abundance of localized mitochondria. The breakdown of keratin begins with the cementing material and progresses to the cortex of the hair shaft. In the cortex two types of degradative patterns are produced which are either parallel or vertical to the axis hair shaft. The parallel pattern arises from hyphal separation of the external cortical layers. The vertical pattern is produced by direct hyphal penetration which creates channels that increase in size as the cortex degrades.

Treatment

The infection cannot easily be removed mechanically, although further proliferation of infection can be achieved by avoidance of moisture. Removal generally involves cutting or shaving of the hair, but chemical treatments may be similarly useful. For women some individuals use a fine comb to remove as much of the infection as possible and then they cut or shave their hair. This is then followed by the application of a sublimate solution in 60% alcohol solution to the scalp. Historical treatments have used alcoholic tinctures of heavy metals, such as mercury bichloride. The application of antifungal shampoos such as pyrithione zinc, formaldehyde and salicylic acid is effective against black piedra. Oral therapy with itraconazole or terbinafine also causes nodules to break down over time. Removal of affected hair and treatment with topical agents is also effective and results in very low recurrences rates. However, even in the absence of treatment, spontaneous remission may occur.

Terbinafine has been used in the treatment.

Cosmetic Uses

Black piedra is sometimes cultivated for cosmetic purposes due to social factors that favour a specific hair colour, which makes them more attractive in their society. Several Indian tribes located from Panama have been known to use several methods in order to darken the hair of albino individuals within their community. One of these methods is the cultivation of black piedra for an extensive period of time in the individuals hair. In Malaysia the nodules of black piedra are very attractive and women are encouraged to sleep with their hair buried in the soil to encourage growth of the black nodules.

Similar Taxa

The genus *Piedraia* contains another species known as *Piedraia quintanilhae*, which is more common in chimpanzees than humans. It differs from *P. hortae* in terms of the ascospores do not have any attachments. Another species known as *Trichosporon biegelii* is commonly known to cause white piedra. White piedra is more common in temperate and semitropical climates, such as South America, Asia, Europe, Japan, and parts of the southern United States. Black piedra usually affects scalp hair, whereas white piedra is more commonly found in pubic hair, axillary hair, beards, moustaches, and eyelashes. White piedra affects horses and monkeys, in addition to humans and the nodules are white and brown in colour and can be easily detached from the hair shaft. White piedra is treated by using topical and antifungal agents, but a more effective approach is to use itraconazole therapy. Recent studies have shown that the black, lichen-colonizing fungus, *Xanthoriicola physciae*, is closely related to *P. hortae*.

Tinea Nigra

Tinea nigra is a dark patch of infected skin. It only affects the most surface-level layer of your skin and is not a dangerous condition. It's not very common, but you'll recognize it for the unique effect it has on your skin.

It's most likely to affect your extremities and shows up more often in tropical climates. Tinea nigra is treatable and doesn't usually have long-term effects on your health.

Symptoms of Tinea Nigra

Tinea nigra can show up on your skin as a rough, brown or black patch. You might mistake it for skin cancer because it gets bigger over time. But a visit to your doctor can clear up any confusion. Your dark spot will be different from skin cancer because it will have an odd shape with a noticeably darker border.

If you have tinea nigra on your hands, you might find that its color changes throughout the day. It is reported to vary from a dark color in the morning to a lighter color in the evening. This can be a result of using your hands to carry out activities during the day.

Another distinctive sign of tinea nigra is where it appears. Tinea nigra commonly affects the palms of your hands and the soles of your feet. It can also develop on your neck. Because tinea nigra doesn't cause discomfort, you might have it for years before you actually get it tested.

Causes of Tinea Nigra

This skin infection happens after you come in contact with a fungus called *Hortaea werneckii. Hortaea werneckii* thrives in hypersaline environments or bodies of water with extremely high salt content. For example, the Dead Sea, which is one of the saltiest lakes in the world, is a hypersaline environment.

Tinea nigra has a long incubation period. This means that it doesn't show up immediately after you come in contact with *Hortaea werneckii*. You'll see color changes in your skin at least 2 to 7 weeks after your exposure to the fungus.

You'll find *Hortaea werneckii* in rotten wood, dirt, composted materials, and sewage, which you're likely to step on or touch. The fungus can enter and infect your body through even the smallest cut or opening in your skin.

Many reported cases of tinea nigra come from humid, tropical areas. If you live in any of the following areas, you're more likely to get this skin infection:

- Panama
- Colombia
- Venezuela
- Brazil
- Mexico
- India
- Sri Lanka
- Myanmar
- Polynesia

Tinea nigra is extremely uncommon in Europe and the United States. But it's still possible to get it in one of these places. If you have hyperhidrosis, or excessive sweating, or live near the ocean, your chances of getting tinea nigra can increase.

Prevention of Tinea Nigra

Tinea nigra can be difficult to prevent because of its subtle and unique cause. You should avoid touching *Hortaea werneckii*, especially if you have any open cuts. If you can, you should stay away from the places where it's most often found.

Risks of Tinea Nigra

There are no serious risks or complications that come along with tinea nigra. It's a superficial skin infection that only changes the color and possibly texture of a small area of your skin. It is not dangerous, but you may want to get rid of it for cosmetic purposes.

Treatment of Tinea Nigra

If you think you might have tinea nigra, you should see a dermatologist. Your infection may clear up on its own, but it's not likely.

Your dermatologist will scrape off a sample of the infected area to test whether you have tinea nigra. This is a quick way to confirm that you have tinea nigra and not skin cancer. If your test comes back positive, you can treat your infection with antifungal skin cream.

The antifungal skin cream will clear up your tinea nigra after 2 to 4 weeks of consistent use. Your dermatologist may even scrape the tinea nigra with a scalpel before you start using the antifungal skin cream.

If your infection goes away but your skin still has dark coloring, you can try scrubbing it. You can also apply a keratolytic agent like salicylic acid to soften and moisturize the healed skin.

Tinea nigra is easy to diagnose and treat. If you think you have it, visit your doctor to make sure that it's a harmless skin infection.

Mould Infections of Nails

Fungal nail infections, also known as "onychomycosis," are very common. They may affect up to 14% of the general population. Fungal toenail infections are more common than fungal fingernail infections.

Symptoms

Most fungal nail infections are not serious. However, some people may experience pain or be bothered by the appearance of their nails.

Fungal nail infections may cause nails to become discolored, thick, fragile, or cracked. The nail may also become separated from the nail bed.

People who have fungal toenail infections often have a fungal skin infection on the foot, especially between the toes (commonly called athlete's foot, ringworm on the foot, or tinea pedis).

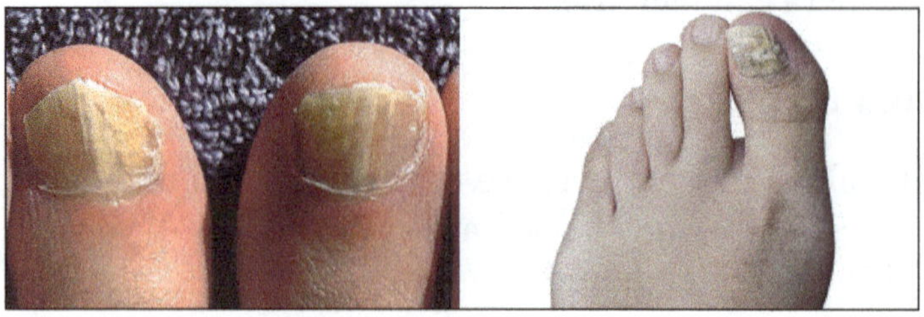

Causes of Fungal Nail Infection

Fungal nail infections are caused by many different types of fungi that live in the environment. Small cracks in your nail or the surrounding skin can allow these germs to enter your nail and cause an infection.

People Susceptible to Fungal Nail Infections

Anyone can get a fungal nail infection. Some people may be more likely than others to get a fungal nail infection, including older adults and people who have the following conditions:

- A nail injury or foot deformity.
- Trauma.
- Diabetes.
- Weakened immune system (for example, because of cancer).
- Venous insufficiency (poor circulation in the legs) or peripheral arterial disease (narrowed arteries reduce blood flow to the arms or legs).
- Fungal skin infections on other parts of the body.

Occasionally, a bacterial infection can occur on top of a fungal nail infection and cause serious illness. This is more common in people with diabetes or other conditions that weaken the body's defenses against infection.

Prevention

- Keep your hands and feet clean and dry.
- Keep fingernails and toenails short and clean.
- Don't walk barefoot in areas like locker rooms or public showers.
- Don't shares nail clippers with other people.
- When visiting a nail salon, choose a salon that is clean and licensed by your state's cosmetology board. Make sure the salon sterilizes its instruments (nail clippers, scissors, etc.) after each use, or bring your own.

Diagnosis

Fungal infections are not the only possible cause of nail problems. Other conditions can look similar to fungal nail infections.

Your healthcare provider should generally confirm your diagnosis using laboratory testing before prescribing antifungal treatment. To confirm the diagnosis, the healthcare provider might collect a nail clipping to look at under a microscope or to send to a laboratory for testing.

Treatment

Fungal nail infections can be difficult to cure, and treatment is most successful when started early. Fungal nail infections typically don't go away on their own, and the best treatment is usually prescription antifungal pills taken by mouth. In severe cases, a healthcare professional might remove the nail completely. It can take several months to a year for the infection to go away.

Fungal nail infections can be closely associated with fungal skin infections. If a fungal infection is not treated, it can spread from one place to the other. Patients should discuss all skin concerns with their healthcare provider to ensure that all fungal infections are properly treated.

Even after treatment, fungal nail infections can come back. This is more common in people who have conditions like diabetes that make them more likely to get a fungal nail infection. If you suspect an infection has returned, contact your healthcare provider.

Information for Healthcare Professionals

Diagnosis

Onychomycosis can be difficult to diagnose based on physical appearance and clinical history alone. Clinicians should confirm a diagnosis of onychomycosis by laboratory testing before prescribing antifungal medications. The following types of laboratory tests can confirm the diagnosis of onychomycosis:

- Microscopy: Potassium hydroxide (KOH) stain can be performed in the office setting, but the accuracy of the test depends on clinician experience and technique. Nail clippings or scrapings are placed in a drop of KOH and examined under a microscope for the presence of fungal elements.
- Histopathologic examination with a periodic acid-Schiff (PAS) stain: Examination of nail clippings with a PAS stain can confirm the diagnosis of a fungal nail infection.
- Culture: Fungal culture can be used to identify the infecting organism, but the fungi may take several weeks to grow.
- Molecular: Molecular testing, including polymerase chain reaction (PCR) testing, may be used to diagnose fungal nail infections.

Antimicrobial-resistant onychomycosis is a growing problem. Therefore, antifungal susceptibility testing may be considered based on the fungus or fungi identified and the patient's clinical course.

Treatment

Oral antifungal therapy should be prescribed only after confirmation of fungal infection. Oral terbinafine is typically the first-line treatment for confirmed onychomycosis. The treatment course is generally 6 weeks for fingernails and 12 weeks for toenails. Given increasing reports of terbinafine resistance in onychomycosis, the possibility of resistance should be considered if patients do not improve with therapy. Identification and susceptibility testing of the causative fungus or fungi may help guide therapy. Note, however, that antimicrobial resistance is not the only possible reason for treatment failure. Clinicians should also consider the possibility of incorrect diagnosis or inadequate patient adherence to therapy.

Topical antifungal agents can be used but are often ineffective. Systemic azoles can also be used. Surgical debridement or removal of the affected nail is also a consideration for cases that are resistant to antifungals, and laser treatments for onychomycosis appear to be a promising area for future study.

Recurrence is common among patients with onychomycosis. To minimize recurrence, clinicians should educate patients about prevention methods (e.g., keeping hands and feet clean and dry) and early signs of disease. Patients should also be aware of the association between onychomycosis and tinea pedis and promptly seek treatment for other tinea lesions.

Invasive Candidiasis

Candidiasis is infection by *Candida* species (most often *C. albicans*), manifested by mucocutaneous lesions, fungemia, and sometimes focal infection of multiple sites. Symptoms depend on the site of infection and include dysphagia, skin and mucosal lesions, blindness, vaginal symptoms (itching, burning, discharge), fever, shock, oliguria, renal shutdown, and disseminated intravascular coagulation. Diagnosis is confirmed by histopathology and cultures from normally sterile sites. Treatment is with amphotericin B, fluconazole, echinocandins, voriconazole, or posaconazole.

Candida species are commensal organisms that inhabit the gastrointestinal (GI) tract and sometimes the skin (see etiology of mucocutaneous candidiasis). Unlike other systemic mycoses, candidiasis results from endogenous organisms. Most infections are caused by *C. albicans*; however, *C. glabrata* (formerly *Torulopsis glabrata*) and other non-albicans species are increasingly involved in fungemia, urinary tract infections, and, occasionally, other focal disease. *C. glabrata* is frequently less susceptible to fluconazole than other species; *C. krusei* is inherently resistant to fluconazole; frequency of resistance to voriconazole and amphotericin varies. *C. krusei* is most frequently susceptible to echinocandins. *C. auris* is an emerging, multidrug-resistant species that has caused recent outbreaks in hospitals and is challenging to identify and treat.

Candida species account for about 80% of major systemic fungal infections and are the most common cause of fungal infections in immunocompromised patients. Candidal infections are one of the most common hospital-acquired infections. Because resistance and transmission of C. auris in health care facilities have become a concern, special infection control precautions have been instituted for patients who are colonized or infected with *C. auris*.

Candidiasis of the esophagus is a defining opportunistic infection in AIDS. Although mucocutaneous candidiasis is frequently present in HIV-infected patients, hematogenous dissemination is unusual unless other specific risk factors are present.

Candida Esophagitis

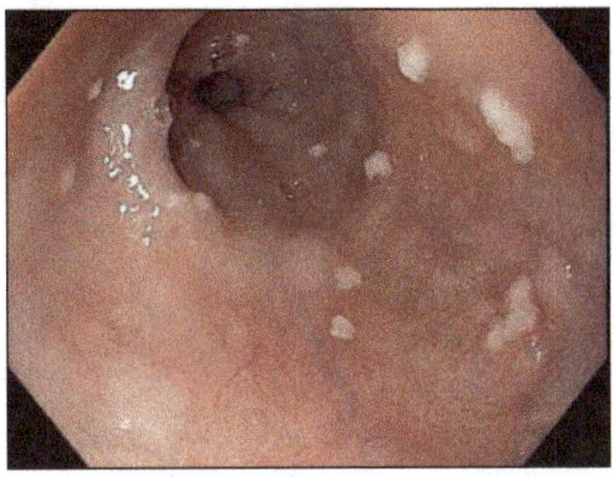

Diffuse whitish plaques are typical of Candida esophagitis.

Candidiasis (Oral)

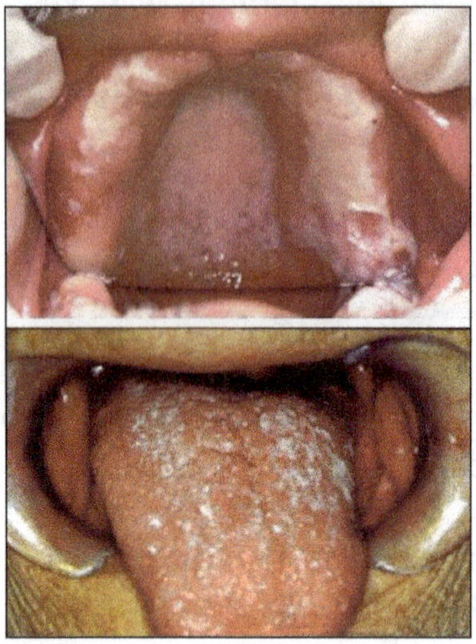

Oral candidiasis takes many forms, including angular cheilitis and pseudomembranous plaques on the oral mucosae, which can be associated with dentures, as in this image (top), or develop on the tongue (bottom) or pharynx.

Oral Candidiasis (Labial Mucosa)

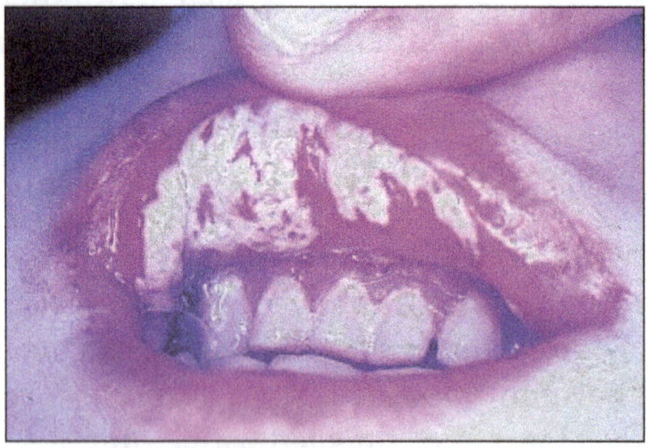

This photo shows oral candidiasis manifesting as a white exudate overlying a beefy, red, and raw mucosal surface of the labial mucosa.

Oral Candidiasis Due to HIV

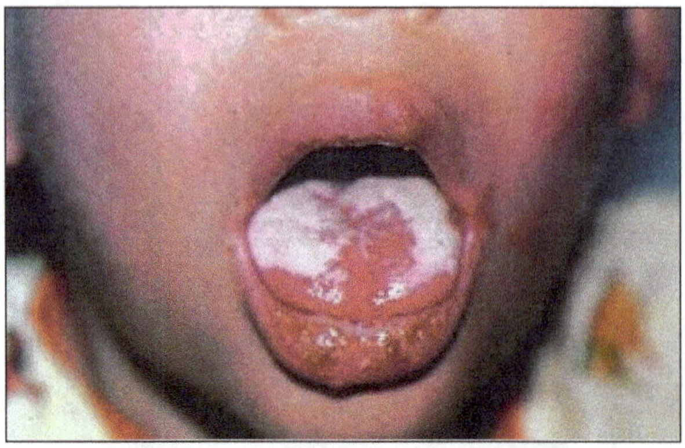

This photo shows fluffy white exudate on the tongue of an HIV-infected child.

Disseminated Candidiasis

Neutropenic patients (eg, complicating cancer chemotherapy) are at high risk of developing life-threatening disseminated candidiasis.

Candidemia may occur in nonneutropenic patients during prolonged hospitalization. This bloodstream infection is often related to one or more of the following:

- Central venous catheters.
- Major surgery.
- Broad-spectrum antibacterial therapy.
- IV hyperalimentation.

IV lines and the GI tract are the usual portals of entry.

Candidemia often prolongs hospitalization and increases mortality due to concurrent disorders. Candidemia may occur with other forms of invasive candidiasis, such as endocarditis or meningitis, as well as focal involvement of skin, subcutaneous tissues, bones, joints, liver, spleen, kidneys, eyes, and other tissues. Endocarditis is commonly related to IV drug abuse, valve replacement, or intravascular trauma induced by indwelling IV catheters.

All forms of disseminated candidiasis should be considered serious, progressive, and potentially fatal.

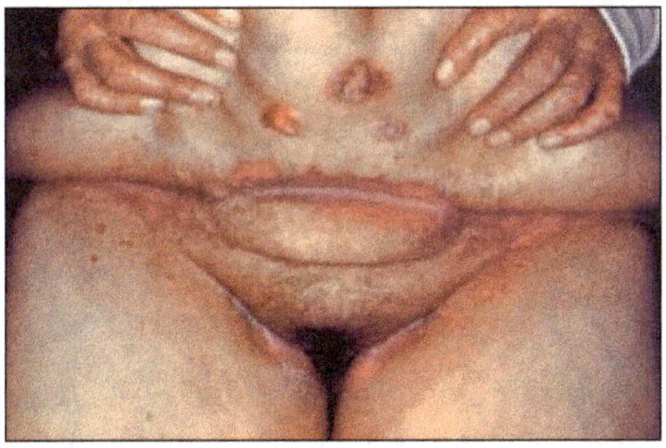

Candidiasis Infection of the Intertriginous Areas of Abdomen and Groin.

This photo shows erythema and superficial ulceration in intertriginous areas of abdomen and groin caused by overgrowth of Candida.

Symptoms and Signs of Invasive Candidiasis

Esophageal candidiasis is most often manifested by dysphagia.

Candidemia usually causes fever, but no symptoms are specific. Some patients develop a syndrome resembling bacterial sepsis, with a fulminating course that may include shock, oliguria, renal shutdown, and disseminated intravascular coagulation.

Candidal endophthalmitis starts as white retinal lesions that are initially asymptomatic but can progress, opacifying the vitreous and causing potentially irreversible scarring and blindness. In neutropenic patients, retinal hemorrhages occasionally also occur, but actual infection of the eye is rare.

Papulonodular skin lesions may also develop, especially in neutropenic patients, in whom they indicate widespread hematogenous dissemination to other organs. Symptoms of other focal or invasive infection depend on the organ involved.

Diagnosis of Invasive Candidiasis

- Histopathology and fungal cultures.
- Blood cultures.
- Serum beta-glucan testing.
- T2Candida® Panel.

Because *Candida* species are commensal, their culture from sputum, the mouth, the vagina, urine, stool, or skin does not necessarily signify an invasive, progressive infection. A characteristic clinical lesion must also be present, histopathologic evidence of tissue invasion (eg, yeasts, pseudohyphae, or hyphae in tissue specimens) must be documented, and other etiologies must be excluded. Positive cultures of specimens taken from normally sterile sites, such as blood, cerebrospinal fluid, pericardium, pericardial fluid, or biopsied tissue, provide definitive evidence that systemic therapy is needed.

Serum beta-glucan is often positive in patients with invasive candidiasis; conversely, a negative result indicates low likelihood of systemic infection.

The T2Candida® Panel is a magnetic resonance assay that directly detects 5 *Candida* species (*C. albicans*, *C. tropicalis*, *C. parapsilosis*, *C. krusei*, and *C. glabrata*) in whole blood samples in 3 to 5 hours. It is highly sensitive and has an excellent negative predictive value. Other molecular diagnostic testing is also available, including matrix-assisted laser desorption ionization–time of flight (MALDI-TOF) mass spectrometry and polymerase chain reaction (PCR)-based assays.

Ophthalmologic examination to check for endophthalmitis is recommended for all patients with candidemia.

Standard laboratory techniques often misidentify *C. auris* as *C. haemulonii*, *C. famata*, *C. sake*, or another species. MALDI-TOF mass spectrometry is a more reliable method for correct identification. A nucleic acid-based test also is now available.

Candida Albicans

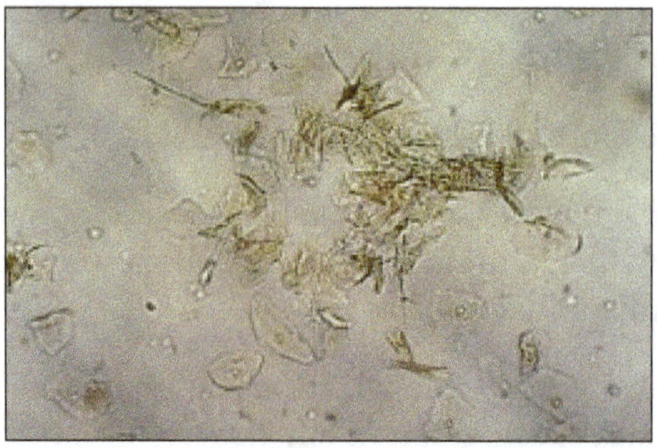

Fungal hyphae or pseudohyphae that are characteristic of Candida albicans can be seen in wet mount preparations.

Treatment of Invasive Candidiasis

- An echinocandin if patients are severely or critically ill or if infection with C. glabrata, C. auris, or C. krusei is suspected.
- Fluconazole if patients are clinically stable or if infection with C. albicans or C. parapsilosis is suspected.
- Alternatively voriconazole or amphotericin B.

Invasive Candidiasis

In patients with invasive candidiasis, predisposing conditions (eg, neutropenia, immunosuppression, use of broad-spectrum antibacterial antibiotics, hyperalimentation, presence of indwelling lines) should be reversed or controlled if possible.

In nonneutropenic patients, IV catheters should be removed.

When an echinocandin is indicated (if patients are moderately severely ill or critically ill [most neutropenic patients] or if *C. glabrata, C. auris*, or *C. krusei* is suspected), one of the following drugs can be used:

- Caspofungin, loading dose 70 mg IV, then 50 mg IV once a day.
- Micafungin 100 mg IV once a day.
- Anidulafungin, loading dose 200 mg IV, then 100 mg IV once a day.

If fluconazole is indicated (if patients are clinically stable or if *C. albicans* or *C. parapsilosis* is suspected), loading dose is 800 mg (12 mg/kg) orally or IV once, followed by 400 mg (6 mg/kg) once a day.

If there is intolerance, limited availability, or resistance to other antifungal drugs, a lipid formulation of amphotericin B at a dosage of 3 to 5 mg/kg IV once a day can be used.

Treatment of invasive candidiasis is continued for 14 days after the last negative blood culture.

Esophageal Candidiasis

Esophageal candidiasis is treated with one of the following:

- Fluconazole 200 to 400 mg orally or IV once a day.
- Itraconazole 200 mg orally once a day.

If these drugs are ineffective or if infection is severe, one of the following may be used:

- Voriconazole 4 mg/kg orally or IV 2 times a day.
- Posaconazole 400 mg orally 2 times a day.
- Isavuconazole 400 mg on day 1, then 100 mg once a day or 200 mg on day 1, then 50 mg once a day or 400 mg once a week.

- An echinocandin.

Treatment of esophageal candidiasis is continued for 14 to 21 days.

Chromoblastomycosis

Chromoblastomycosis is a specific type of cutaneous infection caused by one of several species of dematiaceous (pigmented) fungi. Symptoms are ulcerating nodules on exposed body parts. Diagnosis is by appearance, histopathology, and culture. Treatment is with itraconazole, another azole, or flucytosine **and surgical excision.**

Chromoblastomycosis is a cutaneous infection affecting normal, immunocompetent people mostly in tropical or subtropical areas; it is characterized by formation of papillomatous nodules that tend to ulcerate.

Chromoblastomycosis often occurs at the site of penetrating injury, particularly in farmers and other agricultural workers without adequate protective footwear and clothing.

Chromoblastomycosis is caused by dark brown or black fungi that produce sclerotic bodies in tissue.

Symptoms and Signs of Chromoblastomycosis

Usually, chromoblastomycosis begins on the foot or leg, but other exposed body parts may be infected, especially where the skin is broken. Early small, itchy, enlarging papules may resemble dermatophytosis (ringworm). These papules extend to form dull red or violaceous, sharply demarcated patches with indurated bases. Several weeks or months later, new lesions, projecting 1 to 2 mm above the skin, may appear along paths of lymphatic drainage. Hard, dull red or grayish cauliflower-shaped nodular projections may develop in the center of patches and, if the infection is untreated, gradually extend to cover extremities over the course of many years. Lymphatics may be obstructed, itching may persist, and secondary bacterial superinfections may develop, causing ulcerations and occasionally septicemia.

Chromoblastomycosis (Early)

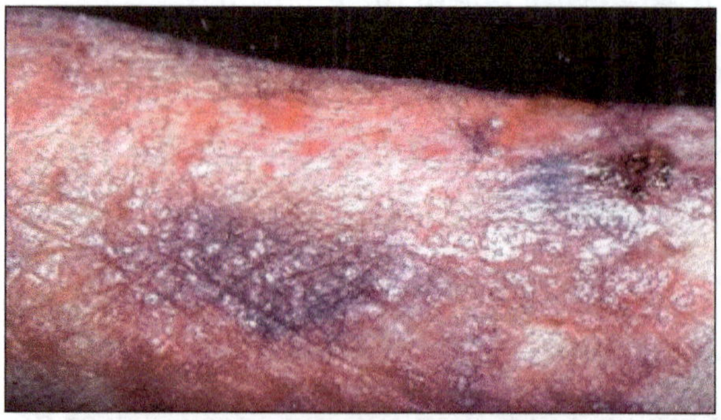

In chromoblastomycosis, small papules initially extend to form dull red or violaceous, sharply demarcated patches with indurated bases.

Chromoblastomycosis (Chronic)

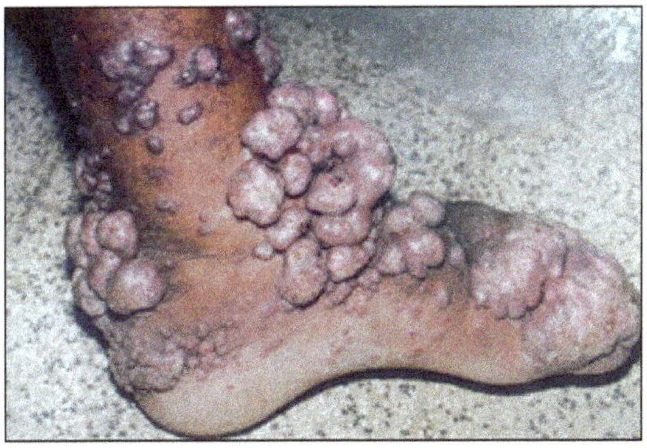

In chronic chromoblastomycosis, hard, dull, red or grayish, cauliflower-shaped nodular projections develop over years and extend to cover the extremities.

Diagnosis of Chromoblastomycosis

- Histopathology
- Culture

Late chromoblastomycosis lesions have a characteristic appearance, but early lesions may be mistaken for dermatophytoses.

Fontana-Masson staining for melanin helps confirm the presence of the sclerotic bodies (Medlar bodies), which are pathognomonic. Culture is needed to identify the causative species.

Treatment of Chromoblastomycosis

- Itraconazole, sometimes with flucytosine.
- Often surgery or cryotherapy.

Itraconazole is the most effective drug for chromoblastomycosis, although not all patients respond. Flucytosine is sometimes added to prevent relapse. Amphotericin B is ineffective. Anecdotal reports suggest that posaconazole, voriconazole, or terbinafine may also be effective.

Adjunctive therapies such as cryotherapy are often helpful, although response is slow.

For localized lesions, surgical excision may be curative.

Lobomycosis

Lobomycosis is a fungal infection of the skin. It usually presents with bumps in the skin, firm swellings, deep skin lesions, or malignant tumors.

It is caused by Lacazia loboi (formerly named Loboa loboi). Transmission is generally by direct contact with contaminated water, soil, vegetation, or by direct contact with an infected dolphin.

Diagnosis is by identifying Lacazia laboi in a lesion.

This disease is usually found in humans and bottlenose dolphins, with the possible risk of transmission from one species to the other.

It was discovered by Brazilian dermatologist Jorge Lobo. Other names which were given to the disease are: keloidal blastomycosis, Amazonian blastomycosis, blastomycoid granuloma, miraip and piraip. These last two names were given by natives of the Amazon and mean that which burns.

Signs and Symptoms

The disease is endemic in rural regions in South America and Central America.Infection most commonly develops after minor scratches or insect bites, but many patients cannot recall any skin trauma. Human-to-human transmission does not occur, and the disease is only acquired from the environment. The disease manifests as chronic keloidal nodular lesions on the ears, legs, or arms.

Diagnosis of Lobo's disease is made by taking a sample of the infected skin (a skin biopsy) and examining it under the microscope. Lacazia loboi is characterized by long chains of spherical cells interconnected by tubules. The cells appear to be yeast-like with a diameter of 5 to 12 μm. Attempts to culture L. loboi have so far been unsuccessful.

Diagnosis

Differential Diagnosis

The disease is often misdiagnosed as Blastomyces dermatitidis or Paracoccidiodes brasiliensis due to its similar morphology.

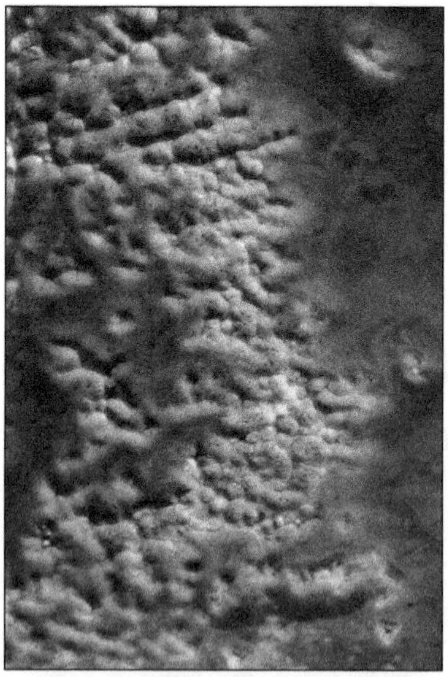

Lobomycosis lesions on the skin of a bottlenosed dolphin.

Treatment

Surgical excision or cryosurgery is the treatment of choice. Treatment with antifungals has been considered ineffective, but the use of clofazimine and dapsone in patients with leprosy and lobomycosis has been found to improve the latter. This treatment regimen, with concomitant itraconazole, has been used to prevent recurrence after surgery.

Mycetoma

Mycetoma is a chronic, progressive local infection caused by fungi or bacteria and involving the feet, upper extremities, or back. Symptoms include tumefaction and formation of sinus tracts. Diagnosis is clinical, confirmed by microscopic examination of exudates and culture. Treatment includes antimicrobials, surgical debridement, and sometimes amputation.

Bacteria, primarily Nocardia species and other actinomycetes, cause more than half the cases. The remainder are caused by about 20 different fungal species. When caused by fungi, the lesions are sometimes called eumycetoma.

Mycetoma occurs mainly in tropical or subtropical areas, including the southern US. Mycetoma occurs in equatorial regions of Africa, Latin America, and Asia known as the "mycetoma belt." Fungal mycetoma (also known as eumycetoma) is the most common type in Africa. Bacterial mycetoma (sometimes referred to as actinomycetoma) causes most cases in South and Central America and some Asian countries.

Mycetoma is acquired when organisms enter through sites of penetrating local trauma on bare skin of the feet or on the extremities or backs of workers carrying contaminated vegetation or other objects. Men aged 20 to 40 are most often affected, presumably because of trauma incurred while working outdoors.

Infections spread through contiguous subcutaneous areas, resulting in tumefaction and formation of multiple draining sinuses that exude characteristic grains of clumped organisms. Microscopic tissue reactions may be primarily suppurative or granulomatous depending on the specific causative agent. As the infection progresses, bacterial superinfections can develop.

Symptoms and Signs of Mycetoma

The initial lesion of mycetoma may be a papule, a fixed subcutaneous nodule, a vesicle with an indurated base, or a subcutaneous abscess that ruptures to form a fistula to the skin surface. Fibrosis is common in and around early lesions. Tenderness is minimal or absent unless acute suppurative bacterial superinfection is present.

Infection progresses slowly over months or years, gradually extending to and destroying contiguous muscles, tendons, fascia, and bones. Neither systemic dissemination nor symptoms and signs suggesting generalized infection occur. Eventually, muscle wasting, deformity, and tissue destruction prevent use of affected limbs. In advanced infections, involved extremities appear grotesquely swollen, forming a club-shaped mass of cystic areas. The multiple draining and intercommunicating sinus tracts and fistulas in these areas discharge thick or serosanguineous exudates containing characteristic grains, which may be white or black.

Manifestations of Mycetoma

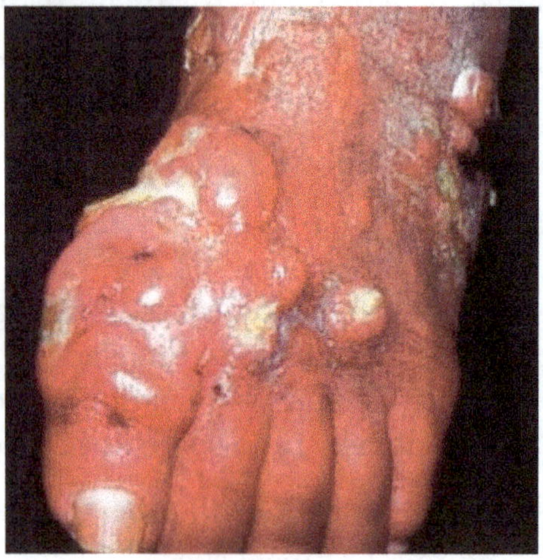

Mycetoma (Nodular).

This image shows multiple, infiltrated nodules on the foot of a patient with mycetoma.

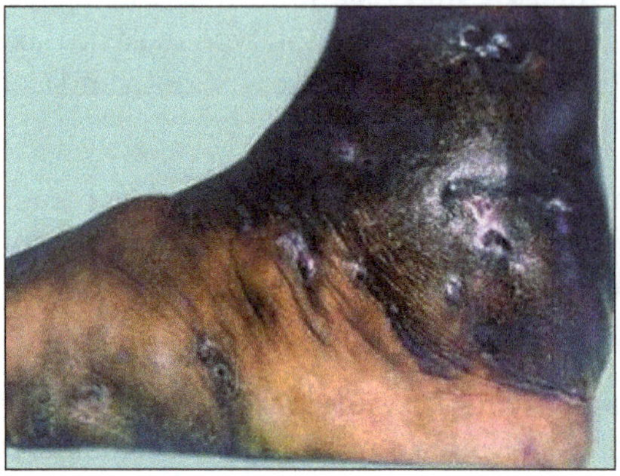

Madura Foot.

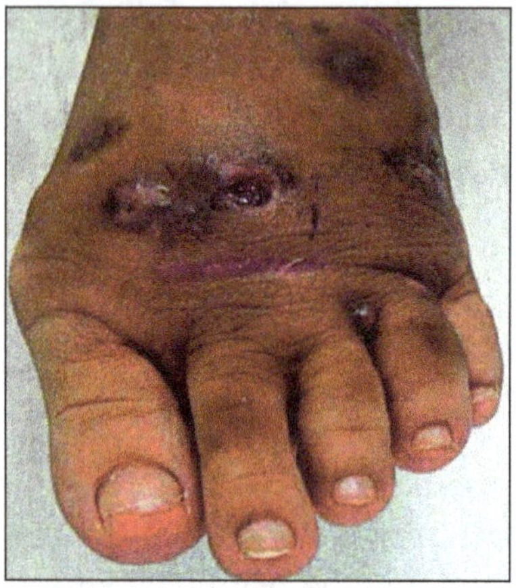

Mycetoma (Skin Rupture).

This image shows multiple subcutaneous nodules and rupture to the skin surface.

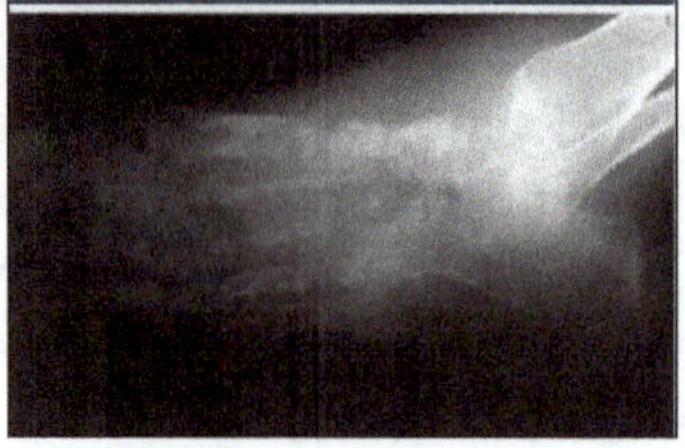

Mycetoma (Madura Foot).

This photo shows chronic, non-healing wounds with recurring episodes of drainage and ulceration (top) and advanced destruction of the entire bony architecture of the foot (bottom).

Diagnosis of Mycetoma

- Examination and culture of exudates.

Causative agents can be identified presumptively by gross and microscopic examination of grains from exudates, which contain pathognomonic, irregularly shaped, variably colored, 0.5- to 2-mm granules. Crushing and culture of these granules provides definitive identification. Exudate specimens may yield multiple bacteria and fungi, some of which are potential causes of superinfections.

Treatment of Mycetoma

- Antibacterial or antifungal drugs.
- Surgery in refractory cases.

Treatment of mycetoma may be required for > 10 years. Death may result from bacterial superinfection and sepsis if treatment is neglected. Treatment depends on the causative agent and the extent of the disease.

In infections caused by Nocardia, sulfonamides and certain other antibacterial drugs, sometimes in combination, are used.

In infections caused by fungi, certain potential causative organisms may be at least partially sensitive to amphotericin B, itraconazole, or ketoconazole, but some are resistant to all antifungal drugs. Relapses occur after antifungal therapy is stopped in most patients, and many patients do not improve and even worsen during treatment, indicating the often refractory nature of the infection.

Surgical debridement is occasionally necessary. Repeated debridement of the diseased tissue, including bone, may be required. Limb amputation to prevent potentially fatal severe secondary bacterial infections may be needed in advanced cases.

Chapter 4

Other Types of Fungal Infections

Cryptococcosis

Most HIV-associated cryptococcal infections are caused by *Cryptococcus neoformans*, but occasionally *Cryptococcus gattii* is the cause. *C. neoformans* is found worldwide, whereas *C. gattii* most often is found in Australia and similar subtropical regions and in the Pacific Northwest. Before the era of effective antiretroviral therapy (ART), approximately 5% to 8% of patients with HIV in high-income countries had disseminated cryptococcosis. In a surveillance study in the late 1990s, people with HIV who developed cryptococcosis were severely immunosuppressed and had limited access to routine HIV medical care. Current estimates indicate that every year, approximately 280,000 cases of cryptococcal infection in people with AIDS occur worldwide, and the disease accounts for 15% of AIDS-related deaths. Overall, 90% of cryptococcal cases in people with HIV are observed in those who have CD4 T lymphocyte (CD4) cell counts <100 cells/mm^3. The incidence of the disease has declined substantially among people treated with ART.

Clinical Manifestations

In people with HIV, cryptococcosis commonly presents as a subacute meningitis or meningoencephalitis with fever, malaise, and headache slowly developing over many weeks, with a median onset of 2 weeks after infection. Classic meningeal symptoms and signs—such as neck stiffness and photophobia—occur in only one-quarter to one-third of patients. Some patients experience encephalopathic symptoms—such as lethargy, altered mentation, personality changes, and memory loss—that are usually a result of increased intracranial pressure (ICP). Among people presenting with cryptococcal meningitis shortly after initiating ART, the symptom onset can be more acute, likely related to unmasking immune reconstitution inflammatory syndrome (IRIS).

Cryptococcosis usually is disseminated when diagnosed in a patient with HIV. In spite of widespread disseminated disease, patients with HIV may manifest few symptoms suggesting a disseminated infection. Any organ can be involved, and skin lesions may show different manifestations, including umbilicated skin lesions that mimic those seen with molluscum contagiosum. Isolated pulmonary infection is also possible; symptoms and signs include cough and dyspnea in association with an abnormal chest radiograph, which typically demonstrates lobar consolidation, although nodular infiltrates have been reported. Pulmonary cryptococcosis may present as acute respiratory distress syndrome and even mimic *Pneumocystis* pneumonia.

Diagnosis

Analysis of cerebrospinal fluid (CSF) generally demonstrates mildly elevated protein levels, low-to-normal glucose concentrations, and a variable presence of pleocytosis consisting mostly of lymphocytes. Some patients with HIV have very few CSF inflammatory cells. A Gram stain or an India ink preparation, if available, may demonstrate numerous yeast forms. In patients with HIV and cryptococcal meningitis, the opening pressure in the CSF may be elevated, with pressures ≥25 cm H_2O occurring in 60% to 80% of patients.

Cryptococcal disease can be diagnosed by culture, CSF microscopy, cryptococcal antigen (CrAg) detection, or CSF polymerase chain reaction (PCR). In patients with HIV-related cryptococcal meningitis, approximately 50% of blood cultures will be positive, and approximately 80% of CSF cultures will be positive. Visible *Cryptococcus* colonies on a Sabouraud dextrose agar plate generally can be detected within 7 days. *Cryptococcus* may be identified occasionally on a routine Gram stain preparation of CSF as poorly staining Gram-positive yeasts. India ink staining of CSF demonstrates encapsulated yeasts in 60% to 80% of cases, but many laboratories in the United States no longer perform this test. India ink is relatively insensitive early in disease when <1,000 *Cryptococcus* colony-forming units (CFU)/mL are present.

CSF CrAg is usually positive in patients with cryptococcal meningoencephalitis; however, early meningitis can present with negative CSF studies and positive CrAg in blood only. Thus, serum CrAg testing always should be performed in an immunocompromised individual with an unknown central nervous system (CNS) disorder. Serum CrAg is positive in both meningeal and non-meningeal cryptococcal infections and may be present weeks to months before symptom onset.

Three methods exist for antigen detection: latex agglutination, enzyme immunoassay (EIA), and lateral flow assay (LFA). The IMMY CrAg LFA (IMMY, Norman, Oklahoma) is the only LFA test for CrAg approved by the Food and Drug Administration (FDA). It is a useful initial screening tool to diagnose cryptococcosis in patients with HIV when applied to serum or plasma, and it also can be used with whole blood or CSF. CrAg testing of serum or plasma may be particularly useful when a lumbar puncture is delayed or refused. In a patient with HIV, when serum CrAg LFA titers are >1:160, disseminated disease becomes increasingly more likely, and when CrAg LFA titers are >1:640, disseminated and/or CNS involvement should be assumed, regardless of CSF test results. Antigen titers by the LFA are approximately fourfold higher than those with latex agglutination or EIA testing, thus a titer of 1:640 by LFA is approximately equal to a titer of 1:160 by EIA or latex agglutination.

In 2016, the BioFire FilmArray Meningitis/Encephalitis Panel PCR assay (Biofire Diagnostics, Salt Lake City, UT) was approved by the FDA. This multiplex PCR tests for 14 targets, including *C. neoformans* and *C. gattii,* and performs well in infections with a moderate to high fungal burden. False negative results have been noted to occur when there is a low burden of organisms; in one study, when there were <100 CFU/mL, the sensitivity of the PCR test fell to 50%. In one well-described case, a woman who had two negative results with this PCR assay later had a positive result on a CrAg test done by IMMY LFA. Thus, a negative CSF PCR does not completely exclude cryptococcal meningitis, and CrAg testing of CSF and blood should always be performed simultaneously. The PCR assay appears to have diagnostic utility when a second episode of cryptococcal meningitis is suspected; the test has been noted to differentiate a relapse (PCR positive) from IRIS (PCR negative).

Preventing Exposure

Cryptococcus is ubiquitous in the environment. People with HIV cannot completely avoid exposure to *C. neoformans* or *C.gattii*.Limited epidemiological evidence suggests that exposure to dried bird droppings, including those from chickens and pet birds, may increase the risk of infection.

Disease Prevention

The incidence of cryptococcal disease is low among people with HIV in the United States. However, one report indicates that among study participants with HIV in the United States with peripheral blood CD4 counts ≤100 cells/mm³, the prevalence of cryptococcal antigenemia—a harbinger of disease—was 2.9%, and for those with CD4 counts ≤50 cells/ mm³, the prevalence was 4.3%. Routine surveillance testing for serum CrAg in people with newly diagnosed HIV who have no overt clinical signs of meningitis is recommended for patients whose CD4 counts are ≤100 cells/mm³ and particularly in those with CD4 counts ≤50 cells/mm³(AII). A positive test generally should prompt CSF evaluation for CNS infection (BIII), particularly when the serum LFA titer is ≥1:160 (AII).

Prospective, controlled trials indicate that prophylactic fluconazole or itraconazole can reduce the frequency of primary cryptococcal disease in patients with HIV who have CD4 counts <100 cells/ mm³. However, in the United States, primary prophylaxis in the absence of a positive serum CrAg test is not recommended because of the relative infrequency of cryptococcal disease, lack of survival benefit associated with prophylaxis, possibility of drug–drug interactions, potential development of antifungal drug resistance, and costs (BII).

Disease Treatment

Treatment consists of three phases: induction, consolidation, and maintenance.

Induction Treatment

For induction treatment of cryptococcal meningitis and other forms of extrapulmonary cryptococcosis, an amphotericin B formulation given intravenously, in combination with oral flucytosine, is recommended (AI). Historically, amphotericin B deoxycholate at a dose of 0.7 to 1.0 mg/kg daily has been the preferred formulation of the drug. However, evidence that lipid formulations of amphotericin B are effective for cryptococcosis is growing, particularly in patients who experience clinically significant kidney dysfunction during therapy or who are likely to develop acute kidney injury. A study that compared amphotericin B deoxycholate (0.7 mg/kg daily) and liposomal amphotericin B (AmBisome®) at two doses (3 mg/kg daily and 6 mg/kg daily) showed similar efficacy for all three regimens; however, less nephrotoxicity was observed among those receiving the 3 mg/ kg daily liposomal amphotericin B regimen. Additional data from animal models and a phase 2 trial in humans, show that single-dose liposomal amphotericin B at a dose of 10 mg/kg has similar rates of CSF yeast clearance and less toxicity than 14 days of amphotericin B deoxycholate.

The preferred regimen for primary induction therapy for patients with normal renal function is 2 weeks of an amphotericin B formulation once daily plus flucytosine 25 mg/kg four times daily (AI). Based on available clinical trial data and clinical experience, liposomal amphotericin B, at a dose of 3 to 4 mg/kg daily, is the favored formulation (AI).

Amphotericin B deoxycholate at a dose of 0.7 to 1.0 mg/kg daily is equally effective and can be used if the costs of lipid formulations are prohibitive and/or interruption of induction therapy because of kidney damage is unlikely (AI).

The noncomparative CLEAR study demonstrated a 58% response rate in patients with HIV who were treated with amphotericin B lipid complex at a mean dose of 4.4 mg/kg daily. Thus, amphotericin B lipid complex at a dose of 5 mg/kg daily can be used as an alternative amphotericin B formulation although fewer data are available to support its use (BII).

When using flucytosine, therapeutic drug monitoring should be performed, if available, particularly in patients who have renal impairment. Serum peak concentrations of flucytosine, should be obtained 2 hours postdose after three to five doses have been administered. Peak serum concentrations should be between 25 mg/L and 100 mg/L. Renal function should be monitored closely and the flucytosine dose adjusted accordingly for patients with renal impairment. The dose of flucytosine should be reduced by 50% for every 50% decline in creatinine clearance. The addition of flucytosine to the amphotericin B regimen during acute treatment is associated with more rapid sterilization of CSF and survival benefit. A randomized clinical trial also showed that the combination of amphotericin B deoxycholate at a dose of 1 mg/kg daily plus flucytosine was associated with improved survival compared to the same dose of amphotericin B without adjunctive flucytosine. Adjunctive fluconazole 800 to 1,200 mg per day plus amphotericin B has been used in the absence of flucytosine, but adjunctive flucytosine has a survival advantage over adjunctive fluconazole and is preferred (AI). Amphotericin B deoxycholate alone or with fluconazole at a dose of 800 to 1,200 mg daily (BI) or lipid-formulation amphotericin B alone (BI) or with fluconazole at a dose of 800 to 1,200 mg daily (BIII) may be viable options in some circumstances, but they are less preferable alternatives than lipid-formulation amphotericin B plus flucytosine.

Fluconazole (1,200 mg daily) plus flucytosine is also a potential alternative to amphotericin B regimens (BII). Some experts would use 800 mg fluconazole daily with flucytosine (BIII). Fluconazole alone, based on studies assessing early fungicidal activity, is inferior to amphotericin B for induction therapy and is recommended only for patients who cannot tolerate or who do not respond to standard treatment. If fluconazole alone is used for primary induction therapy, the starting daily dose should be 1,200 mg (CI).

The duration of induction therapy historically has been 2 weeks. In a multicenter clinical trial that evaluated 10-week outcomes of treatment of cryptococcal meningitis in 721 African adults with HIV, 1 week of amphotericin B deoxycholate therapy was shown to be noninferior to 2 weeks, and at 1 year, follow-up of 236 patients from this treatment trial showed continued noninferiority of the 1-week regimen compared with the 2-week regimen. Thus, in resource-limited settings, 1 week of amphotericin B deoxycholate with flucytosine followed by high-dose fluconazole is now preferred (BIII). However, in high-resource settings where the less toxic liposomal or other lipid amphotericin B formulations is used and a greater capacity to provide supportive care to mitigate amphotericin B toxicities exists, 2 weeks of induction amphotericin B combination therapy is recommended (AI).

Consolidation Treatment

A lumbar puncture and repeat CSF culture should be performed after 2 weeks of induction therapy. At that point, clinically stable patients may be switched to consolidation therapy while awaiting CSF culture results. Successful induction therapy is defined as substantial clinical improvement and a negative CSF culture from the end-of-induction lumbar puncture. India ink and CSF CrAg frequently remain positive at Week 2 of therapy and are not indicative of failure. Monitoring serum or CSF CrAg titers is of no value in determining initial response to therapy and is not recommended (AII). If new symptoms or clinical findings occur later, a repeat lumbar puncture, with measurement of lumbar opening pressure and CSF culture, should be performed.

Consolidation therapy should be initiated with fluconazole 800 mg daily (AI). The recommendation to use 800 mg rather than 400 mg fluconazole for consolidation therapy is based on several findings. Early clinical trials that used 400 mg fluconazole for consolidation noted breakthrough infection during consolidation. Fluconazole 400 mg per day provides concentrations in the CSF that are only fungistatic, and other studies showed that the early antifungal activity of fluconazole in CSF of patients with cryptococcal meningitis increases linearly with increasing doses of the drug. A phase 2 trial of treatment with either 400 mg or 800 mg fluconazole found that relapses were more frequent in patients receiving 400 mg fluconazole. In clinically stable patients, the dose of fluconazole for consolidation therapy should be 800 mg per day until CSF cultures are known to be sterile and ART is initiated, at which point the dose can be decreased to 400 mg per day (AII).

For patients who have completed 2 weeks of induction therapy, but have not improved clinically or remain clinically unstable, continuation of amphotericin B plus flucytosine is recommended until the CSF cultures are confirmed to be negative (BIII). For patients who have improved clinically, but whose CSF remains culture positive after 2 weeks of induction therapy, the fluconazole dose should be increased to 1,200 mg per day and another lumbar puncture should be performed 2 weeks later (BIII). For all patients with CSF cultures positive at Week 2, the duration of consolidation therapy should be 8 weeks from the time the CSF cultures are negative (AI).

An alternative approach for outpatients who are not ill enough to be hospitalized but still have positive CSF cultures after completing 2 weeks of induction therapy is to continue flucytosine for an additional 2 weeks together with fluconazole at a dose of 1,200 mg per day before starting single-drug consolidation therapy.

Itraconazole can be used as an alternative therapy for consolidation (CI), but it is clearly inferior to fluconazole. Limited data are available for use of the newer triazoles—voriconazole, posaconazole, and isavuconazole—for either consolidation or maintenance therapy for patients with cryptococcosis. Most of the reported data have been on use of these extended-spectrum triazole antifungals for treatment of refractory cases, with success rates of approximately 50%. Currently, the role of posaconazole, voriconazole, and isavuconazole in the initial management of cryptococcosis has not been established in randomized clinical trials, and these agents are not recommended for consolidation or maintenance therapy (AIII). Echinocandins have no activity against *Cryptococcus* spp. and are not recommended for clinical management of cryptococcosis (AII).

Maintenance Treatment

Fluconazole 200 mg per day is used for maintenance treatment and continue until at least one year from initiation of antifungal therapy (AI).

Treatment of Non-CNS Cryptococcosis and Asymptomatic Antigenemia

Non-CNS, extrapulmonary cryptococcosis and diffuse pulmonary disease should be treated the same as CNS disease (BIII). For those with mild to moderate symptoms and only focal pulmonary infiltrates, treatment with fluconazole 400 to 800 mg per day for 10 weeks followed by 200 mg daily for a total of 6 months combined with effective ART is recommended (BIII).

Patients with isolated or asymptomatic cryptococcal antigenemia without meningitis and low serum CrAg titers (i.e., <1:320 using LFA) can be treated in a similar fashion as patients with mild to moderate symptoms and only focal pulmonary cryptococcosis with fluconazole 400 to 800 mg per day (BIII). If the serum CrAg titer by LFA is ≥1:640 (or >1:160 by EIA or latex agglutination), even in the absence of meningitis, the risk for mortality and/or progression to meningitis increases with fluconazole monotherapy alone, and patients should be treated the same as patients with cryptococcal meningitis (BIII). All patients with asymptomatic cryptococcal antigenemia should have their CSF sampled to rule out CNS disease. If serum CrAg titers are >1:640 with the LFA test and a CSF sample is not available, CNS involvement should be assumed regardless of CSF culture results or clinical signs or symptoms, and the patient should be treated as detailed above for CNS disease (AII).

Special Considerations with Regard to Starting ART

Unlike with other opportunistic infections, ART initiation generally is deferred for 4 to 6 weeks after antifungal agents are started (AI). A randomized clinical trial conducted at three sites in Africa compared patients with cryptococcal meningitis who started ART within 1 to 2 weeks (median 8 days) after the diagnosis of meningitis with patients for whom ART was delayed for 4 to 6 weeks (median 35 days) after diagnosis. This clinical trial used amphotericin B deoxycholate 0.7 to 1.0 mg/kg once daily plus fluconazole 800 mg once daily during the induction phase of antifungal treatment. A significantly greater increase in 6-month mortality occurred in the early ART group than in the delayed ART group (45% versus 30%, $P = 0.03$). This increase was most pronounced during the first 8 to 30 days of study ($P = 0.007$). The difference in mortality between the early ART group and the delayed ART group was even greater among individuals with CSF white cell count <5 cells/μL ($P = 0.008$). The excess of deaths in the early ART group was likely attributable to paradoxical IRIS.

Most experts aim to start ART after 4 to 6 weeks of antifungal therapy; however, individual patient factors may alter this timing. In general, ensuring that the patient's CSF cultures are sterile before starting ART will reduce the risk of IRIS. If ART must be started sooner, the patient should be monitored closely for paradoxical IRIS with a low threshold to intervene. For non-CNS cryptococcosis, for which the risk of IRIS appears to be lower, the optimal time to begin ART and antifungal therapy is less clear. However, in patients with non-CNS cryptococcosis, it is prudent to delay initiation of ART for 2 weeks after starting antifungal therapy (BIII).

All of the triazole antifungals have the potential for complex and possibly bidirectional interactions with certain antiretroviral agents. These interactions and recommendations for dosage adjustments, where feasible, are listed in the drug–drug interaction tables in the Guidelines for the Use of Antiretroviral Agents in Adults and Adolescents with HIV.

Monitoring of Response to Therapy and Adverse Events

Elevation of ICP can cause clinical deterioration despite a microbiologic response; complications are more likely to occur if the CSF lumbar opening pressure is ≥25 cm H_2O in the lateral decubitus position. In a large clinical trial in patients with AIDS and cryptococcal meningitis, increased ICP was associated with 93% of deaths during the first 2 weeks of antifungal therapy and 40% of deaths during weeks 3 to 10. In another clinical trial, patients with HIV-associated cryptococcal meningitis who received at least one therapeutic lumbar puncture within 7 days after diagnosis (median time of 3 days) had a 69% relative reduction in the risk of death through 11 days, regardless of initial opening pressure. Although it is uncertain which patients with high lumbar opening pressures will experience clinical deterioration, those with symptoms and signs of increased ICP require immediate clinical intervention to reduce ICP.

Control of elevated ICP is critical to reducing acute mortality. Lumbar opening pressure should be measured in all patients with cryptococcal meningitis at the time of diagnosis. However, in routine practice, CSF opening pressure frequently is not measured. Among patients in whom CSF opening pressure was not measured initially, a repeat lumbar puncture should be performed with measurement of opening pressure. For patients with ongoing headaches, a repeat lumbar puncture should be performed with urgency, and among those without headaches, a repeat lumber puncture should be considered strongly within 48 hours of the initial procedure. Measures to decrease ICP should be used for all patients with confusion, blurred vision, papilledema, lower extremity clonus, or other neurologic signs indicative of increased ICP. Drainage of CSF via lumbar puncture is recommended for initial management (AII). One approach is to remove a volume of CSF that at least halves the opening pressure or normalizes the pressure to <20 cm H_2O. In the absence of a manometer, removal of 20 to 25 mL of CSF is recommended (AIII). Among patients with ongoing symptoms, therapeutic lumbar punctures should be repeated daily until symptoms and signs consistently improve and opening pressure normalizes to <20 cm H_2O (AII). Because a survival benefit is associated with therapeutic lumbar puncture regardless of baseline CSF opening pressure, strong consideration should be given to repeating a therapeutic lumbar puncture within 72 hours of the initial procedure in those patients who are relatively asymptomatic or who had a baseline CSF opening pressure of <20 cm H_2O, (BII). This second lumbar puncture can be especially useful if the initial opening pressure was not measured (AII). ICP can be a dynamic process that changes over time.

CSF shunting through a lumbar drain or ventriculostomy should be considered for patients who cannot tolerate repeated lumbar punctures or for those in whom signs and symptoms of increased ICP persist after multiple lumbar punctures (BIII). Corticosteroids and mannitol have been shown to be ineffective in managing ICP and are not recommended (AIII). Acetazolamide should not be used as therapy for increased ICP management because it may exacerbate hyperchloremic acidosis from amphotericin B and does not result in a decrease in ICP (AI). A randomized study that compared a 6-week course of a tapering dose of dexamethasone with placebo among 451 Asian and African patients with cryptococcal meningitis found that dexamethasone did not improve survival through 10 weeks, was noted to decrease killing of *Cryptococcus,* and was associated with more adverse events. These data support the recommendation that corticosteroids should not be used during induction therapy for ICP control for HIV-associated cryptococcal meningitis unless they are being used for treatment of IRIS (AI).

Patients treated with amphotericin B formulations should be monitored for nephrotoxicity and electrolyte disturbances. Pre-infusion administration of 1,000 mL of normal saline reduces the risk of nephrotoxicity during amphotericin B treatment. For people with severe infusion-related adverse reactions, acetaminophen (650 mg) and diphenhydramine (25–50 mg) or hydrocortisone (50–100 mg) typically are administered 30 minutes before the infusion to reduce the severity of amphotericin infusion reactions (CIII), but scant data exist to support these practices. Meperidine (25–50 mg titrated during infusion) is effective for preventing and treating amphotericin B–associated rigors (BII). Routine use of potassium chloride, 40 mEq per day and magnesium 8 mEq per day, supplementation should be considered because the risk of hypokalemia and hypomagnesemia becomes near universal after 1 week of therapy, regardless of amphotericin B formulation (AII).

In patients receiving flucytosine, dosage should be adjusted based on changes in creatinine clearance and can be guided by flucytosine levels. Peak serum flucytosine levels should be obtained 2 hours after an oral dose; the therapeutic range is between 25 and 100 mg/L. If therapeutic drug monitoring is not possible or kidney dysfunction is not present, frequent complete blood counts with differential (i.e., at least biweekly) can be used to detect cytopenias (BII). Flucytosine is associated with concentration-dependent bone marrow toxicity. Patients treated with flucytosine also should be monitored for hepatotoxicity and gastrointestinal toxicities.

Common side effects of higher dose fluconazole therapy can include dry skin (17% of patients) and alopecia (16% of patients). Increased liver transaminases or alkaline phosphatase are relatively rare with fluconazole 400 to 800 mg use, with only 1 to 2% having values >5 times the upper limit of normal. For people who have difficulty tolerating higher fluconazole doses, it appears safe to reduce the consolidation therapy fluconazole dose to 400 mg per day after initiation of ART (BII).

Immune Reconstitution Inflammatory Syndrome

An estimated 10 to 30% of people with HIV who have cryptococcal meningitis experience IRIS after initiation or re-initiation of effective ART. Patients with HIV who have cryptococcal IRIS are more likely to be ART naive and have less CSF inflammation on initial presentation. The risk of IRIS can be minimized by achieving CSF culture sterility before starting ART, using fluconazole 800 mg per day as consolidation therapy, and deferring ART initiation for 4 to 6 weeks from the start of antifungal therapy (AII). Distinguishing paradoxical IRIS from treatment failure with culture-positive relapse is difficult. In general, cryptococcal IRIS presents with worsening clinical disease despite microbiological evidence of effective antifungal therapy with sterile CSF cultures, whereas treatment failure is associated with continued positive cultures. The primary microbiological criterion for treatment failure is a CSF culture that yields *Cryptococcus*; the culture may take days to weeks to become positive. A negative PCR test (e.g., Biofire FilmArray Meningitis/Encephalitis Panel) has a high predictive value for predicting sterile CSF cultures and can be diagnostically useful to distinguish paradoxical IRIS with a negative CSF PCR from culture-positive relapse with a positive CSF PCR.

The appropriate management strategy for IRIS is to continue both ART and antifungal therapy and reduce elevated ICP if present (AII). While diagnostic tests are pending, escalating antifungal therapy is appropriate, such as restarting amphotericin B therapy or increasing the fluconazole dose to 1,200 mg per day (BIII). In patients with severe symptoms of IRIS, some experts recommend a brief course of tapering doses of corticosteroids. Dosages have varied, but commonly start at 1.0 mg/kg per day of prednisone (BIII); precise data-driven management strategies have not been developed. Serum C–reactive protein (CRP) is generally elevated at the time IRIS develops; CRP will decrease with corticosteroid therapy if IRIS is present and can be used to monitor IRIS resolution. At hospital discharge, restarting fluconazole therapy at consolidation therapy doses to be continued for 8 weeks is recommended (BIII).

The risk of IRIS appears to be much lower and the syndrome seems to be less severe with other forms of cryptococcosis—such as lymphadenitis, cutaneous abscesses, and bony lesions—than with cryptococcal meningitis. Management of IRIS with other forms of cryptococcosis is similar to that for IRIS associated with cryptococcal meningitis, including continuing ART, initiating or continuing antifungal therapy (AIII), and considering the use of corticosteroids if clinical symptoms are severe (CIII).

Managing Treatment Failure

Treatment failure is defined as: (1) a lack of clinical improvement and continued positive cultures after 2 weeks of appropriate therapy that has included management of increased ICP, or (2) relapse after an initial clinical response, defined as recurrence of symptoms with a positive CSF culture after ≥4 weeks of treatment. Primary fluconazole resistance in *Cryptococcus* isolates has been reported in the United States but is uncommon. Therefore, susceptibility testing is not recommended routinely for initial management of cryptococcosis. However, if treatment failure or relapse occurs, *Cryptococcus* isolates should undergo antifungal susceptibility testing. Robust clinical data are lacking, but strains of *Cryptococcus* with fluconazole minimum inhibitory concentrations (MIC) ≥16 µg/mL are considered not fully susceptible.

Optimal therapy for patients with treatment failure has not been established. Patients who do not respond to induction with fluconazole monotherapy should be switched to amphotericin B, with or without flucytosine. Those initially treated with an amphotericin B formulation should remain on this agent until clinical response occurs. In this setting, liposomal amphotericin B (4–6 mg/kg daily) or amphotericin B lipid complex (5 mg/kg daily) is better tolerated and has greater efficacy than the deoxycholate formulation and should be considered when initial treatment with other regimens fails (AII).

In the setting of treatment failure or relapse, verifying CSF culture sterility at the completion of re-induction therapy is critical (AIII). After CSF sterility is achieved, outpatient consolidation therapy should consist of fluconazole at a higher dose of 1,200 mg per day and optimization of ART. For *Cryptococcus* with decreased azole-susceptibility (i.e., >16 µg/mL MIC for fluconazole) some experts would recommend adjunctive weekly amphotericin B administration during consolidation therapy (BIII). Higher doses of fluconazole (i.e., 1,200 mg per day) in combination with flucytosine 25 mg/kg 4 times per day also may be considered (BI). The newer triazoles—posaconazole, voriconazole, and isavuconazole—have activity against *Cryptococcus* spp. *in vitro* and may have a role in salvage therapy, but they offer no specific advantages over fluconazole unless *in vitro* susceptibility testing indicates high-level fluconazole resistance. Most clinical failures are not due to antifungal drug resistance, but rather result from inadequate induction therapy, nonadherence, drug interactions that decrease the serum concentrations of fluconazole (e.g., with rifampin), or the development of paradoxical IRIS.

Preventing Recurrence

Starting of Maintenance Therapy

Patients who have completed 10 weeks of induction and consolidation therapy for cryptococcal meningitis or disseminated cryptococcosis should be treated with chronic maintenance or suppressive therapy with fluconazole 200 mg per day for at least 1 year (AI). Itraconazole is inferior to fluconazole for preventing relapse of cryptococcal disease (CI). One study demonstrated that only 70% of patients receiving fluconazole 200 mg per day achieved therapeutic concentrations of fluconazole in plasma when the fluconazole MIC was >8 μg/mL, and only 30% when the MIC was 16 μg/mL. For patients in whom susceptibility studies have been performed and the fluconazole MIC is >8 μg/mL, some experts recommend that the fluconazole dose be increased to 400 mg per day (BIII). Failure to administer secondary prophylaxis for an entire year is the most common reason for subsequent relapse of cryptococcal disease.

Termination of Maintenance Therapy

Only a few patients have been evaluated for relapse after successful antifungal therapy for cryptococcosis and discontinuation of maintenance therapy while on ART. In a European study, recurrences of cryptococcosis were not found among 39 participants on potent ART whose antifungal therapy was discontinued. In this cohort, when maintenance therapy was stopped, the median CD4 count was 297 cells/mm^3, the median HIV RNA concentration was <500 copies/mL, and the median time on potent ART was 25 months. A prospective, randomized study of 60 patients in Thailand documented no recurrences of cryptococcosis during 48 weeks of follow-up among 22 patients whose antifungal therapy was discontinued after reaching a CD4 count >100 cells/mm^3 with a sustained undetectable HIV RNA level for 3 months on potent ART. Given these data and inference from data on discontinuation of secondary prophylaxis for other HIV-associated opportunistic infections, it is reasonable to discontinue maintenance therapy after at least 1 year from initiation of antifungal therapy, in patients whose CD4 counts are >100 cells/mm^3 with undetectable viral loads on ART (BII). Maintenance therapy should be reinitiated if the CD4 count decreases to <100 cells/mm^3(AIII).

Special Considerations during Pregnancy

The diagnosis of cryptococcal infections in individuals who are pregnant is similar to that in individuals who are not pregnant. Treatment should be initiated promptly after a diagnosis is confirmed. It should be emphasized that initiating antifungal therapy during the postpartum period is associated with an increased risk of IRIS.

Lipid formulations of amphotericin B are preferred for the initial regimen for the treatment of cryptococcal meningoencephalitis, disseminated disease, or severe pulmonary cryptococcosis in patients who are pregnant. Extensive clinical experience with amphotericin B has not documented teratogenicity. Neonates born to women on chronic amphotericin B at delivery should be evaluated for renal dysfunction and hypokalemia.

In animal studies, flucytosine is teratogenic; experience in humans is limited to case reports and small series. Therefore, flucytosine use should be considered only when the benefits outweigh the risks to the fetus and only in the third trimester (AIII).

Fluconazole is teratogenic in the first trimester. Congenital malformations similar to those observed in animals exposed to the drug—including craniofacial and limb abnormalities—have been reported in infants born to mothers who received fluconazole at doses of ≥400 mg per day through or beyond the first trimester of pregnancy. A recent systematic review and meta-analysis of cohort or case-control studies reporting fetal outcomes after exposure to fluconazole in the first trimester of pregnancy analyzed more than 16,000 exposures and found an association with increased risk of heart defects and spontaneous abortion; exposure to a fluconazole dose ≥150 mg was associated with an increase in overall congenital malformations. One registry-based cohort study included in the systematic review and a more recent large population-based case-control study specifically noted an increase in conotruncal heart defects. The latter study also suggested an increase in cleft lip with cleft palate.

A nationwide cohort study in Denmark also found that exposure to oral fluconazole during pregnancy was associated with an increased risk of spontaneous abortion compared with unexposed pregnancies or those with topical azole exposure only. A cohort study using Swedish and Norwegian registry data (n = 1,485,316 pregnancies) found no association between fluconazole use during pregnancy and risk of stillbirth or neonatal death. Most of the studies regarding effects of fluconazole during pregnancy have involved low doses of the drug and short-term exposure.

On the basis of reported birth defects, the FDA classified fluconazole as pregnancy category D for any use other than a single dose of fluconazole 150 mg to treat vaginal candidiasis. Use of fluconazole in the first trimester should be considered only if the benefits clearly outweigh the risks. For pregnant women, amphotericin B should be continued throughout the first trimester. After induction therapy, weekly amphotericin B has been used for consolidation therapy for women who are pregnant throughout the first trimester. After the first trimester, switching to oral fluconazole 200 mg per day may be considered if appropriate clinically.

In a case series of 12 pregnant Ugandan women with cryptococcal meningitis who received amphotericin B deoxycholate 0.7 to 1 mg/kg induction therapy, maternal mortality was 25%. Stillbirths and miscarriages were common during the initial maternal hospitalization with only 33% (4 live births out of 12 pregnancies) fetal survival. Consolidation therapy comprised weekly amphotericin during the first trimester and fluconazole thereafter. With life-threatening cryptococcal disease, fetal demise is common even without fluconazole exposure.

Although case reports of birth defects in infants exposed to itraconazole exist, prospective cohort studies of >300 women with first-trimester exposure did not show an increased risk of fetal malformation. However, in general, azole antifungals should be avoided during the first trimester of pregnancy (BIII). Voriconazole (at doses lower than recommended human doses), posaconazole, and isavuconazole are teratogenic and embryotoxic in animals; no adequately controlled studies have assessed their teratogenicity and embryotoxicity in humans. Voriconazole, posaconazole, and isavuconazole are not recommended for use during pregnancy, especially in the first trimester (AIII).

Mucormycosis

Mucormycosis is a type of fungal infection. It's relatively rare, but also very serious.

Formally known as zygomycosis, this infection tends to occur most often if you have weakened immunity from an illness or health condition.

It's important to get treatment. If left untreated, mucormycosis can be fatal.

Pictures of Mucormycosis

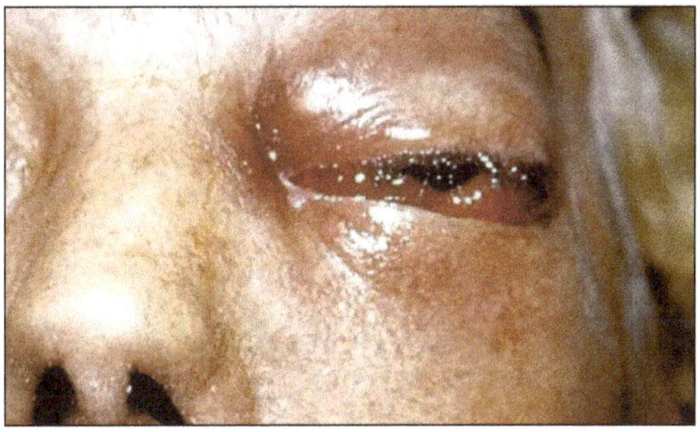

Symptoms of Mucormycosis

Mucormycosis presents itself as either a respiratory or a skin infection. Signs of a related sinus or respiratory infection may include:

- Cough.
- Fever.
- Headache.
- Nasal congestion.
- Sinus pain.

With a skin infection, mucormycosis can develop within any part of your body. It may initially occur at the site of skin trauma, but it can quickly spread to another area. Be on the lookout for symptoms such as:

- Blackened skin tissue.
- Blisters.
- Fever.
- Redness.
- Swelling.

- Tenderness.
- Ulcers.

Causes of Mucormycosis

Mucormycosis is caused by exposure to mucormyete molds. These organisms occur in:

- Leaves.
- Piles of compost.
- Soil.
- Rotting wood.

You can contract mucormycosis by breathing in affected mold spores in the air. This is referred to as a sinus (pulmonary) exposure. In turn, you may develop the infection in your:

- Central nervous system (rarer).
- Eyes.
- Face.
- Lungs.
- Sinuses.

The fungus can also infect your skin via a cut or burn (cutaneous exposure). In such cases, the wound or burn ends up becoming the area of infection.

While these types of molds can naturally occur in the environment, not everyone exposed will get the fungal infection. You may be at an increased risk of contracting this type of infection if you have a weakened immune system. Conditions that may increase your risk include:

- Burns.
- Cuts and scrapes.
- Cancer.
- Recent organ transplant.
- HIV or AIDS.
- Diabetes (especially if it's not being treated properly).
- Surgery.

Ways of Diagnosing Mucormycosis

People who have mucormycosis often don't know they have it. You may get diagnosed with the condition upon going to the doctor for a lung, sinus, or skin infection. You should see your doctor for any type of suspected infection.

Mucormycosis is diagnosed by looking at a tissue sample in the lab. Your doctor may collect a sample of phlegm or nasal discharge if you have a suspected sinus infection. In the case of a skin infection, your doctor may also clean the wounded area in question.

Can Mucormycosis cause other Conditions to Develop

Mucormycosis is particularly dangerous because it spreads quickly throughout the body. Left untreated, the infection can spread to the lungs or the brain. This can cause:

- A brain infection.
- Paralysis.
- Pneumonia.
- Seizures.
- Death.

Treatment of Mucormycosis

The first steps in treating mucormycosis are receiving intravenous (IV) antifungal medications and having surgical debridement. Surgical debridement involves cutting away all infected tissue. Removing infected tissue has been shown to prevent the infection from spreading further.

If you respond well to IV therapy and tissue removal, your doctor will likely remove your IV and give you oral medications to take.

Common antifungal medications that your doctor may prescribe for mucormycosis include:

- Amphotericin B (given through an IV).
- Posaconazole (given through an IV or orally).
- Isavuconazole (given through an IV or orally).

Blastomycosis

Blastomycosis, also known as Gilchrist's disease, is a fungal infection, typically of the lungs, which can spread to brain, stomach, intestine and skin, where it appears as crusting purplish warty plaques with a roundish bumpy edge and central depression. Only about half of people with the disease have symptoms, which can include fever, cough, night sweats, muscle pains, weight loss, chest pain, and feeling tired. Symptoms usually develop between three weeks and three months after breathing in the spores. In 25% to 40% of cases, the infection also spreads to other parts of the body, such as the skin, bones or central nervous system. Although blastomycosis is especially dangerous for those with weak immune systems, most people diagnosed with blastomycosis have healthy immune systems.

Blastomyces dermatitidis is found in the soil and decaying organic matter like wood or leaves. Outdoor activities like hunting or camping in wooded areas increase the risk of developing blastomycosis. There is no vaccine, but the risk of the disease can be reduced by not disturbing the soil. Treatment is typically with an azole drug such as itraconazole for mild or moderate disease. In severe cases, patients are treated with amphotericin B before azole treatment. In either event, the azole treatment lasts for 6–12 months. Overall, 4-6% of people who develop blastomycosis die; however, if the central nervous system is involved, this rises to 18%. People with AIDS or on medications that suppress the immune system have the highest risk of death at 25-40%.

Blastomycosis is endemic to the eastern United States and Canada, especially the Ohio and Mississippi River valleys, the Great Lakes, and the St. Lawrence River valley. In these areas, there are about 1 to 2 cases per 100,000 per year. Less frequently, blastomycosis also occurs in Africa, the Middle East, India, and western North America. Blastomycosis also affects a broad range of non-human mammals, and dogs in particular are an order of magnitude more likely to contract the disease than humans. The ecological niche of Blastomyces in the wild is poorly understood, and it is unknown if there are any significant host animals.

Blastomycosis has existed for millions of years but was first described by Thomas Caspar Gilchrist in 1894. Because of this, it is sometimes called "Gilchrist's disease".

Signs and Symptoms

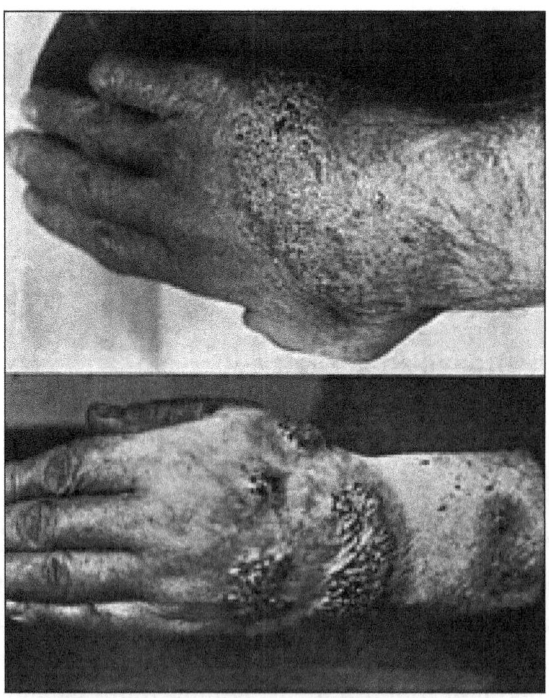

Skin lesions caused by blastomycosis.

The symptoms of blastomycosis cover a wide range, overlapping with more common conditions; for this reason, blastomycosis has often been called "the great pretender". Many cases are asymptomatic or subclinical. Lung symptoms are common, because the lungs are infected in 79% of blastomycosis cases. However, in 25-40% of cases the disease also disseminates to other organs, including the skin.

The extent and severity of symptoms depends in part on a person's immune status; less than 50% of healthy people with blastomycosis have symptoms, while immunocompromised patients are especially likely to have the disease spread beyond the lungs to other organs like the skin and bones.

Blastomycosis manifests as a primary lung infection in about 79% of cases. The onset is relatively slow and symptoms are suggestive of bacterial pneumonia, often leading to initial treatment with antibacterials. Because the symptoms are variable and nonspecific, blastomycosis is often not even considered in differential diagnosis until antibacterial treatment has failed, unless there are known risk factors or skin lesions. The disease may be misdiagnosed as a carcinoma, leading in some cases to surgical removal of the affected tissue. Upper lung lobes are involved somewhat more frequently than lower lobes. If untreated, many cases progress over a period of months to years to become disseminated blastomycosis.

Blastomycosis in the lungs may present a variety of symptoms, or no symptoms at all. If symptoms are present they may range from mild pneumonia resembling a pneumococcal infection to acute respiratory distress syndrome (ARDS). Common symptoms include fever, chills, headache, coughing, difficulty breathing, chest pain, and malaise. Without treatment, cases may progress to chronic pneumonia or ARDS.

ARDS is an uncommon but dangerous manifestation of blastomycosis. It was seen in 9 of 72 blastomycosis cases studied in northeast Tennessee. Such cases may follow massive exposure, such during brush clearing operations. In the Tennessee study, the fatality rate was 89% in the ARDS cases, but only 10% in the non-ARDS cases.

In disseminated blastomycosis, the large Blastomyces yeast cells translocate from the lungs and are trapped in capillary beds elsewhere in the body, where they cause lesions. The skin is the most common organ affected, being the site of lesions in approximately 60% of cases. The signature image of blastomycosis in textbooks is the indolent, verrucous or ulcerated dermal lesion seen in disseminated disease. Osteomyelitis is also common (12–60% of cases). Other recurring sites of dissemination are the genitourinary tract (kidney, prostate, epididymis; collectively ca. 25% of cases) and the brain (3–10% of cases). 40% of immunocompromised individuals have CNS involvement and present as brain abscess, epidural abscess or meningitis.

Blastomycosis in non-lung organs such as the skin may present a very wide range of symptoms, including the following:

- Skin lesions, which may be verrucous (wart-like) or ulcerated with small pustules at the margins.
- Bone or joint pain due to bone lytic lesions.
- Pain when urinating due to prostatitis.
- Hoarseness due to laryngeal involvement.

- Headache, confusion or other neurological symptoms caused by central nervous system involvement.

Cause

Blastomycosis is caused by dimorphic fungi in the genus Blastomyces, in the phylum Ascomycota and family Ajellomycetaceae. In eastern North America, the most common cause of blastomycosis is Blastomyces dermatitidis, but Blastomyces gilchristii has been associated with some outbreaks. In western North America, many cases of blastomycosis are caused by Blastomyces helicus, which most commonly attacks immunodeficient people and domestic animals. The species Blastomyces percursus causes many cases of blastomycosis in Africa and the Middle East. In Africa, blastomycosis may also be caused by Blastomyces emzantsi, which is often associated with infections outside the lungs.

In endemic areas, Blastomyces dermatitidis lives in soil and rotten wood near lakes and rivers. Although it has never been directly observed growing in nature, it is thought to grow there as a cottony white mold, similar to the growth seen in artificial culture at 25 °C. The moist, acidic soil in the surrounding woodland harbors the fungus.

Pathogenesis

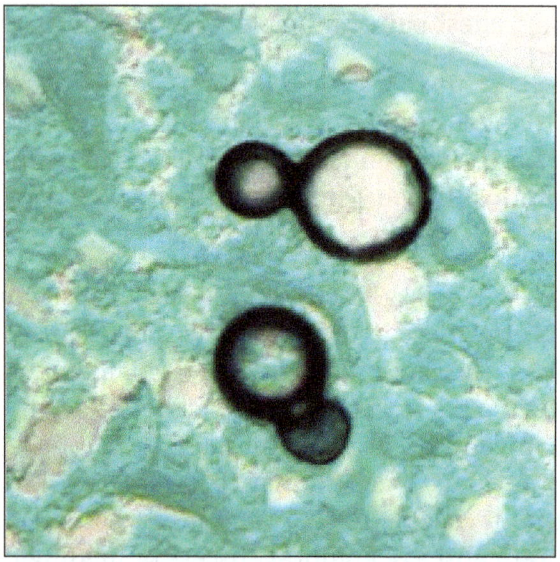

Large, broadly-based budding yeast cells characteristic of Blastomyces dermatitidis in a GMS-stained biopsy section from a human leg.

Inhaled conidia of Blastomyces are phagocytosed by neutrophils and macrophages in alveoli. Some of these escape phagocytosis and transform into yeast phase rapidly. Having thick walls, these are resistant to phagocytosis. Once they have transitioned to the yeast phase, the Blastomyces cells express the protein BAD-1, which helps the yeast cells attach to host cells, and also impairs activation of immune cells while inhibiting release of tumor necrosis factor. In lung tissue, the cells multiply and may also disseminate through blood and lymphatics to other organs, including the skin, bone, genitourinary tract, and brain. The incubation period for pulmonary blastomycosis is 3 to 15 weeks, although 30–50% of infections are asymptomatic.

Diagnosis

Because the symptoms of blastomycosis resemble those of many other conditions, including tuberculosis and lung cancer, diagnosis is often delayed. In 40% of cases, the diagnosis takes more than a month. A rapid diagnosis can however be made based on microscopic examination of sputum samples or samples obtained from a tissue biopsy or bronchoalveolar lavage.

Once suspected, the diagnosis of blastomycosis can usually be confirmed by demonstration of the characteristic broad based budding organisms in sputum or tissues by KOH prep, cytology, or histology. Tissue biopsy of skin or other organs may be required in order to diagnose extra-pulmonary disease. Blastomycosis is histologically associated with granulomatous nodules.

Commercially available urine antigen testing appears to be quite sensitive in suggesting the diagnosis in cases where the organism is not readily detected. However, commercial antigen tests have a high degree of cross-reactivity with other endemic fungal conditions such as histoplasmosis, and thus cannot distinguish blastomycosis from other similar conditions. This cross-reactivity is caused by these related fungal organisms using similar galactomannans in the cell wall.

While culture of the Blastomyces organism remains the definitive diagnostic standard, its slow growing nature can lead to a delay of up to four weeks. In addition, sometimes blood and sputum cultures may not detect blastomycosis. Cultures of the cerebrospinal fluid also have poor sensitivity compared to histopathological examination of the affected tissue.

Treatment

Under Infectious Disease Society of America guidelines, severe cases of blastomycosis and cases with central nervous system (CNS) involvement are treated initially with amphotericin B, followed by a lengthy course of an azole drug such as itraconazole. In most cases the amphotericin treatment lasts for 1–2 weeks, but in cases of CNS involvement it may last for up to 6 weeks. Cases that do not require amphotericin B treatment are treated with a lengthy course of an azole drug.

Among azole drugs, itraconazole is generally the treatment of choice. Voriconazole is often recommended for CNS blastomycosis cases due to its ability to pass the blood–brain barrier. Other azole drugs that may be used include fluconazole. Ketoconazole was the azole drug first used for blastomycosis treatment, but has been largely replaced by itraconazole because ketoconazole is less effective and less tolerated by patients. The azole treatment generally lasts for a minimum of six months. Cure rates from itraconazole treatment are nearly 95%. Relapse is rare but does occur even after a full course of treatment.

Coccidioidomycosis

Meaning of Valley Fever

Valley fever, also called coccidioidomycosis ("cahk-sid-ee-oy-doh-my-KOH-sis"), is an infection caused by breathing in the fungus *Coccidioides* ("cahk-sid-ee-OY-deze"). *Coccidioides* lives in the soil in the southwest U.S., parts of Washington state, and Central and South America. It's named for the San Joaquin Valley in California, where it was first discovered.

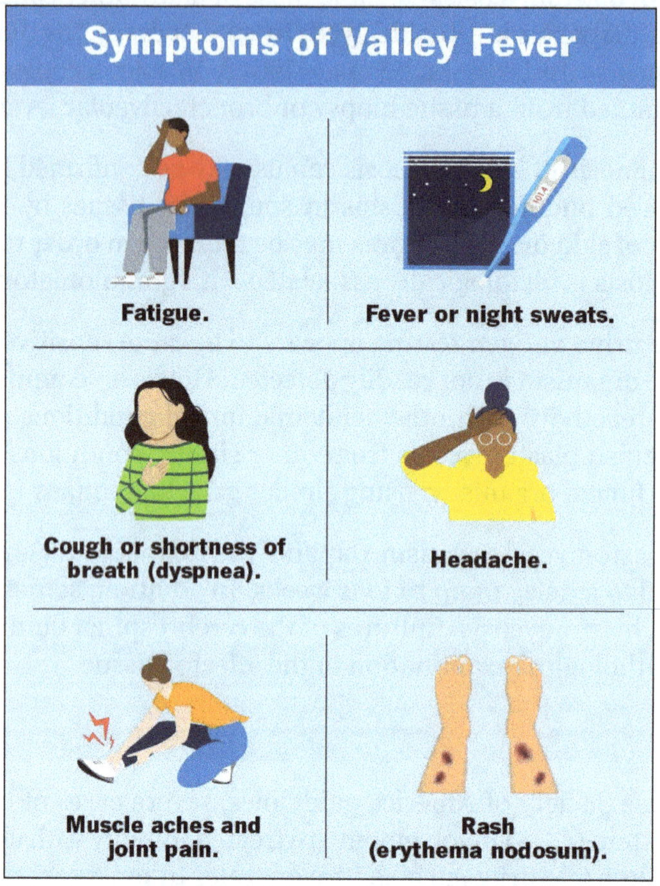

Symptoms of Valley fever are usually mild or flu-like, though most people with Valley fever have no symptoms. Chronic pulmonary coccidioidomycosis causes additional symptoms like coughing up blood, weight loss and chest pain.

Valley fever is the earliest stage of a *Coccidioides* infection. Valley fever often has no symptoms or flu-like symptoms, but it can sometimes progress to more serious stages of coccidioidomycosis.

People those are at Risk of Getting Valley Fever

Anyone who breathes in the fungus can get infected, but Valley fever is most common in adults over age 60.

Certain people are also at higher risk:

- People with weakened immune systems, which can be caused by certain medications or diseases like HIV/AIDS.
- Pregnant people in their third trimester.
- People living with diabetes.
- Blacks and Filipinos.

- People who have jobs that expose them to soil dust.
- Anyone who's recently traveled or moved to an area where the fungus lives.

Places where Valley Fever is Mostly Common

About 20,000 people are diagnosed with Valley fever each year. It's most common in California and Arizona.

Effect of Valley Fever on Body

The *Coccidioides* fungus breaks apart into microscopic reproductive parts (spores) that travel through the air you breathe. They settle into the airways in your lungs where they grow into larger clusters of more spores (spherules).

The spherules can break apart and send more spores out into other parts of your lungs and sometimes other parts of your body. Those spores can grow into spherules of more spores and keep spreading the fungus in your body.

Symptoms and Causes

Symptoms of Valley Fever

In many cases, Valley fever doesn't cause any symptoms. If you do have symptoms of Valley fever, they might include:

- Fatigue.
- Fever or night sweats.
- Cough or shortness of breath (dyspnea).
- Headache.
- Muscle aches and joint pain.
- Rash (erythema nodosum).

When seen together, fever, nodules under the skin and joint stiffness are sometimes called desert rheumatism.

Lasting Period of Valley Fever

Symptoms of Valley fever usually go away on their own after a few weeks or months.

A small number of people can have ongoing disease in their lungs. If it goes on for a long time, it's usually called chronic pulmonary coccidioidomycosis instead of Valley fever. This may be symptomless or cause symptoms like:

- Chronic cough.

- Coughing up blood (hemoptysis).
- Weight loss.
- Chest pain.
- Shortness of breath (dyspnea).

Causes of Valley Fever

There are two forms of *Coccidioides* fungi that cause Valley fever: *Coccidioides immitis* (*C. immitis*) grows in the soil in California and *Coccidioides posadasii* (*C. posadasii*) grows in other parts of the U.S. and Central and South America. They both cause the same symptoms.

Disturbing the soil — particularly during construction or dust storms — breaks apart the fungus, which releases its reproductive parts (spores) into the air. You inhale the spores and they settle in your lungs where they can grow and spread more spores. The spores themselves and your immune system's response to them cause symptoms.

Complications of Valley Fever

Complications of Valley fever are uncommon, with only about 1% of those who are symptomatic going on to develop severe cases. Serious complications include:

- Pneumonia.
- Fluid or pus in your lungs (pleural effusion or empyema).
- Acute respiratory distress syndrome (ARDS).
- Ruptured pockets of fluid or air in your lungs (hydropneumothorax).
- Disease spread outside of your lungs (disseminated coccidioidomycosis).

Disseminated (Extrapulmonary) Coccidioidomycosis

One of the most serious complications of Valley fever is when the fungus spreads outside of your lungs. It can spread to your skin, bones, joints, liver, pancreas, kidneys and brain. When coccidioidomycosis spreads to your brain, you can develop coccidioidal meningitis, a life-threatening condition. Symptoms of coccidioidal meningitis include:

- Headaches.
- Blurred vision.
- Sensitivity to light.
- Neck stiffness.
- Hearing changes.
- Confusion.

Valley fever contagious or not

No, Valley fever isn't contagious from person to person like the flu. In extremely rare cases, you might be able to inhale spores from an open wound on someone who has Valley fever but this is unlikely. Most of the time, the only way to get it is to inhale spores from the air outdoors.

Diagnosis and Tests

Ways of Diagnosing Valley Fever

To diagnose Valley fever, your healthcare provider will perform a physical exam and ask you about your symptoms and travel history. They may order blood tests, imaging (chest X-ray or CT scan) or biopsies.

Tests to Diagnose Valley Fever

To diagnose Valley fever, your healthcare provider may order some or all of these tests:

- Blood tests: Blood tests are the most common way to diagnose Valley fever. Your provider uses a needle to take blood from your vein, which they then send to a lab to look for certain signs of coccidioides (antibodies or antigens).
- Biopsy: Your provider may take a small amount of tissue and send it to a lab to look for signs of coccidioides.
- Imaging: Your provider may use a chest X-ray or CT scan to look for Valley fever pneumonia, a potentially serious complication. This will give your provider pictures of your lungs to see if there are any changes that indicate pneumonia.

Management and Treatment

Treatment of Valley Fever

Treatment for Valley fever will depend on how severe your condition is and how your provider wants to manage it. They might recommend keeping an eye on your symptoms before prescribing medications, or they might treat you in order to reduce the risk of serious illness. If you have a serious or ongoing infection or if you have risk factors for severe illness (like chronic pulmonary disease) they may prescribe antifungal medications.

Medications to Treat Valley Fever

If you need to be treated for Valley fever, your healthcare provider may prescribe one of these medications:

- Fluconazole.
- Itraconazole.
- Amphotericin B (AmB).

Lasting of the Treatment of Valley Fever

Your healthcare provider may prescribe antifungal treatments for Valley fever for three to six months. Your treatment may last longer depending on your case.

Histoplasmosis

Histoplasmosis is a type of lung infection. It is caused by inhaling Histoplasma capsulatum fungal spores. These spores are found in soil and in the droppings of bats and birds. This fungus mainly grows in the central, southeastern, and mid-Atlantic states.

Most cases of histoplasmosis don't require treatment. However, people with weaker immune systems may experience serious problems. The disease may progress and spread to other areas of the body. Skin lesions have been reported in 10 to 15 percent of cases of histoplasmosis that has spread throughout the body.

Things to Look at

Most people who are infected with this fungus have no symptoms. However, the risk of symptoms increases as you breathe in more spores. If you are going to have symptoms, they generally show up about 10 days after exposure.

Possible symptoms include:

- Fever.
- Dry cough.
- Chest pain.
- Joint pain.
- Red bumps on your lower legs.

In severe cases, symptoms may include:

- Excessive sweating.
- Shortness of breath.
- Coughing up blood.

Widespread histoplasmosis causes inflammation and irritation. Symptoms may include:

- Chest pain, caused by swelling around the heart.
- High fever.
- Stiff neck and headaches, from swelling around the brain and spinal cord.

Causes

Fungal spores can be released into the air when contaminated soil or droppings are disturbed. Breathing the spores may lead to an infection.

The spores that cause this condition are commonly found in places where birds and bats have roosted, such as:

- Caves
- Chicken coops
- Parks
- Older barns

You can get histoplasmosis more than once. However, the first infection is generally the most severe.

The fungus doesn't spread from one person to another and it's not contagious.

Types of Histoplasmosis

Acute

Acute, or short-term, histoplasmosis is typically mild. It rarely leads to complications.

The Centers for Disease Control and Prevention (CDC) estimate that between 60 and 90 percent-Trusted Source of people who live in areas where the fungus is common have been exposed. Many of these people probably did not have any symptoms of infection.

Chronic

Chronic, or long-term, histoplasmosis occurs far less often than the acute form. In rare cases, it can spread throughout the body. Once histoplasmosis has spread throughout your body it is life-threatening if it isn't treated.

Widespread disease usually occurs in people with impaired immune systems. In areas where the fungus is common, the CDC says that it may occur in up to 30 percent of people with HIV.

Risk Factors

There are two major risk factors for developing this disease. The first is working in a high-risk occupation and the second risk factor is having a compromised immune system.

Occupations

You are more likely to be exposed to histoplasmosis if your job exposes you to disturbed soil or animal droppings. High-risk jobs include:

- Construction worker.
- Farmer.

- Pest control worker.
- Demolition worker.
- Roofer.
- Landscaper.

Weakened Immune Systems

Many people who have been exposed to histoplasmosis do not get noticeably sick. However, your risk of severe infection is higher if you have a compromised immune system. Conditions associated with weakened immunity include:

- Being very young or very old.
- Having HIV or AIDS.
- Taking strong anti-inflammatory medications like corticosteroids.
- Undergoing chemotherapy for cancer.
- Taking TNF inhibitors for conditions such as rheumatoid arthritis.
- Taking immunosuppressant drugs to prevent a transplant rejection.

Potential Long-Term Complications of Infection

In rare cases, histoplasmosis can be life-threatening. Therefore, it is extremely important to get treatment.

Histoplasmosis can also cause a number of complications.

Acute Respiratory Distress Syndrome

Acute respiratory distress syndrome can develop if your lungs fill with fluid. This can lead to dangerously low levels of oxygen in your blood.

Heart Function Issues

Your heart might not be able to function normally if the area around it becomes inflamed and full of fluid.

Meningitis

Histoplasmosis can cause a serious condition called meningitis. Meningitisoccurs when the membranes surrounding your brain and spinal cord become infected.

Adrenal Glands and Hormone Problems

Infection can damage your adrenal glands and this may cause problems with hormone production.

Testing for and Diagnosing Histoplasmosis

If you have a mild case of histoplasmosis, you may never know that you were infected. Testing for histoplasmosis is usually reserved for people who both have a severe infection and live or work in a high-risk area.

To confirm a diagnosis, your doctor may conduct blood or urine tests. These tests check for antibodies or other proteins that indicate prior contact with histoplasmosis. Your doctor might also take urine, sputum, or blood cultures to make an accurate diagnosis. However, it can take up to six weeks to get results.

Depending on what parts of your body are affected, you may need other tests. Your doctor might take a biopsy(tissue sample) of your lung, liver, skin, or bone marrow. You might also need an X-ray or computerized tomography (CT) scan of your chest. The purpose of these tests is to determine if additional treatments are needed to address any complications.

Treatments for Histoplasmosis

If you have a mild infection, you probably won't need treatment. Your doctor might instruct to you rest and take an over-the-counter medication for symptoms.

If you have trouble breathing or are infected for longer than one month, treatment may be necessary. You will likely be given an oral antifungal medication, but you may also require IV treatment. The most commonly used drugs are:

- Ketoconazole.
- Amphotericin B
- Itraconazole.

If you have a severe infection, you might need to take your medication intravenously (through a vein). This is how the strongest medications are delivered. Some people may have to take antifungal medication for up to two years.

Prevention of Histoplasmosis

You can reduce your risk of infection by avoiding high-risk areas. These include:

- Construction sites.
- Renovated buildings.
- Caves.
- Pigeon or chicken coops.

If you can't avoid high-risk areas, there are steps you can take to help keep spores from getting into the air. For example, spray sites with water before working or digging in them. Wear a respirator mask when there is a high risk of exposure to spores. Your employer is obligated to provide you with appropriate safety equipment if it's needed to protect your health.

Paracoccidioidomycosis

Paracoccidioidomycosis is a rare disease that is caused by a specific fungus.

Paracoccidioidomycosis is a rare tropical disease that is caused by the fungus *Paracoccidioides brasiliensis*. This disease is most common throughout Central and South America and is usually transmitted by a person inhaling spores of the *P. brasiliensis* fungus. (Hugo most likely inhaled this fungus while hiking through the forest.) Most often, paracoccidioidomycosis initially affects the lungs, but it can also spread to other parts of the body, such as the skin. Symptoms usually do not appear until several weeks or months after being infected with the fungus. These symptoms include:

- Cough.
- Shortness of breath.
- Fatigue.
- Chest pain.
- Ulcers on the skin and around the nose and mouth.
- Fever.

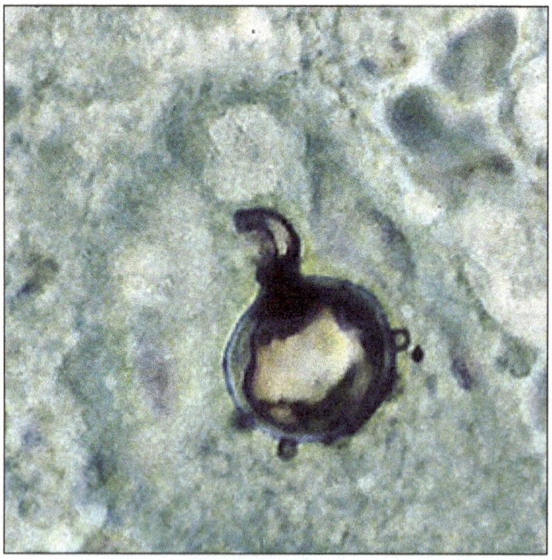

Paracoccidioidomycosis is a disease caused by the Paracoccidioides brasiliensis fungus.

Histology

Histology is the microscopic study of the cells and tissues of animals and plants. In regards to paracoccidioidomycosis, there are many changes that occur to the cells and tissues of an infected person. Lung tissues will often become scarred and fibrotic, which can make the lungs very stiff and breathing very difficult.

These changes can also cause increased blood pressure in the blood vessels in the lungs, leading to a condition called cor pulmonale. Cor pulmonale involves the increase in size of the muscular tissue in the right ventricle, which is the chamber of the heart that pumps blood to the lungs. Since the blood pressure in the lungs has increased, the right ventricle has to work extra hard to pump blood against this pressure, causing the muscles of this ventricle to increase over time.

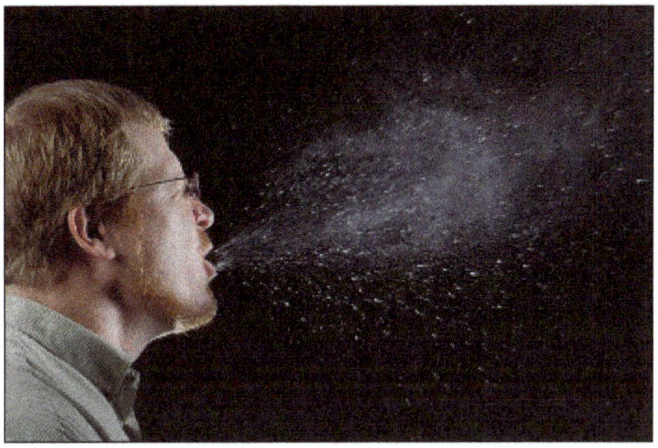

A common symptom of paracoccidioidomycosis is coughing.

Paracoccidioidomycosis can also cause granulomas to form in the cells and tissues of the skin. Granulomas are collections of white blood cells (WBCs) that surround a foreign substance in the body. The role of WBCs is to find and destroy foreign substances in the body, such as fungi. When these WBCs find a fungus, they will surround it, kill it, and eliminate it from the body. However, sometimes they surround a fungus but are not able to eliminate it from the body, which causes a granuloma to form.

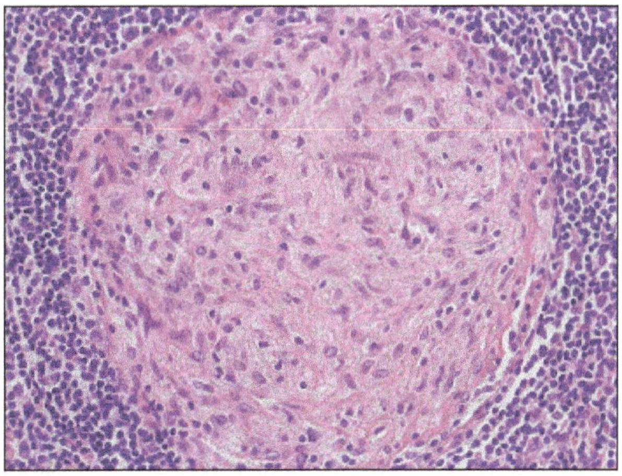

Paracoccidioidomycosis can result in the formation of granulomas in the skin tissue.

Prevention

Unfortunately, there are currently no known vaccines that protect the body against *P. brasiliensis*. One of the best measures of prevention would be to avoid areas where this fungus is commonly found, such as the forests and woods of Central and South America. Additionally, since paracoccidioidomycosis is usually transmitted by inhaling the *P.brasiliensis* fungal spores, this disease can be prevented by wearing simple masks that help block these spores from entering the mouth and lungs.

Rhinofacial Conidiobolomycosis

- Conidiobolomycosis was considered a rare subcutaneous tissue infection.
- Rhinofacial is a primary affected area of conidiobolomycosis.
- It is mostly indolent, chronic process, and non-angioinvasive in nature.
- Early recognition and treatment can prevent organ disfiguration.

Entomophthoramycosis can be found in subtropical and tropical regions. This case illustrates common clinical features of conidiobolomycosis. Although this disease is not common, physicians working in these regions should be familiar with the clinical manifestations to enable early diagnosis and treatment.

A 58-year-old gardener and immunocompetent man presented with a 3-month history of painless bulging, mild erythema, and firm consistency of the right nasal alar, nasolabial area, cheek, and dorsum of the nose. Anterior rhinoscopy revealed firm soft-tissue swelling in the nasal vestibule and head of the inferior turbinate and almost total occlusion of the right nasal cavity. Computed tomographic scans of the paranasal sinuses showed poorly defined infiltrative lesions in the right nasal cavity, nose, and upper lip. Biopsy samples from the right nasal cavity demonstrated intramucosal eosinophilic granulomas with nonseptate fungal hyphae. Culture from the nasal cavity grew hyaline fungi. The patient was diagnosed with conidiobolomycosis. He received itraconazole and potassium iodide and responded well to the treatment.

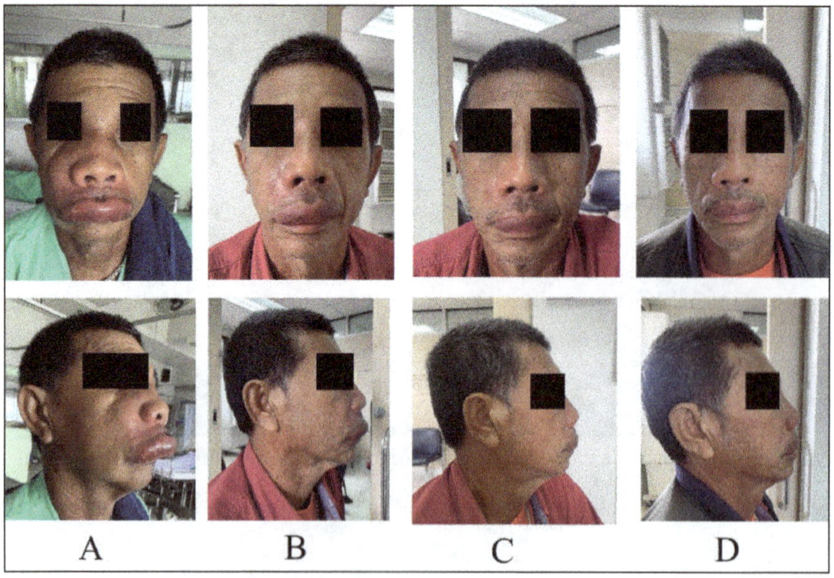

(a) Before treatment; (b) 2 weeks after treatment; (c) 6 weeks after treatment; (d) 1 year after treatment.

Entomophthoramycosis (conidiobolomycosis and basidiobolomycosis) is caused by fungi belonging to the subphylum Entomophthoramycotina. There are no extensive studies on its incidence. Conidiobolomycosis primarily affects the rhinofacial area by an indolent, chronic, and nonangioinvasive process. Patients may acquire the spores of Conidiobolus spp. from either inhalation or direct skin inoculation. Despite indefinite diagnosis in this case, the clinical features, pathologic findings, culture results, and response to the treatment support the diagnosis of conidiobolomycosis. Early recognition and prompt treatment can halt disease progression and prevent disfiguration of the affected organ.

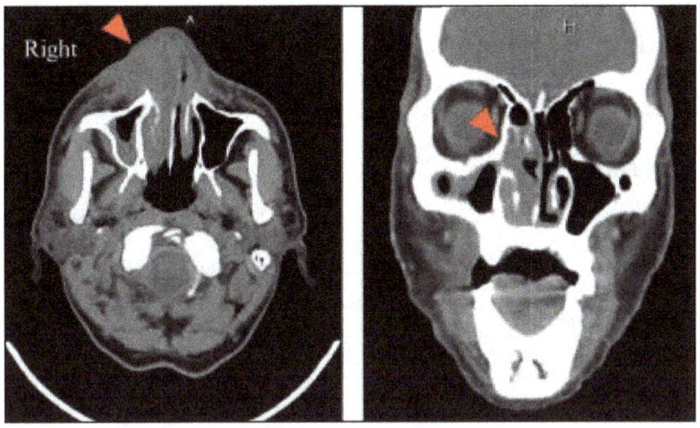

Computed tomographic images of the paranasal sinuses. A: anterior, H: head, Red arrow: ill-defined infiltrative lesions at the right nasal cavity, nose, and upper lip.

Basidiobolomycosis

- Basidiobolomycosis is a rare fungal infection caused by environmental saprophyte Basidiobolus ranarum
- It is a member of the order Entomophthorales of the class zygomycetes
- The zygomycetes include two fungal orders:
    - Mucorales, involving mainly immunocompromised patients, and
    - Entomophthorales, which causes infection in immunocompetent individuals.
- Basidiobolomycosis is endemic in tropical and subtropical regions of Africa, Latin America, Middle East and Asia.
- It mainly involves skin and subcutaneous tissue and rarely infects the gastrointestinal tract.
- First case of visceral basidiobolomycosis (GIB) was reported in 1964.

Essential Features

- Basidiobolomycosis is a rare fungal infection caused by Basidiobolus ranarum.
- Causes infection in immunocompetent individuals.
- Is endemic in tropical and subtropical regions.
- Mainly involves skin and subcutaneous tissue, visceral involvement is rare.
- Infection is caused by ingestion of contaminated food or use of contaminated toilet paper.

- Abdominal pain and fever are most common presenting features.
- Histology shows broad septate thin walled fungal hyphae with the Splendore-Hoeppli phenomenon.
- Culture is gold standard for diagnosis.
- Treatment: combined surgery and medical therapy with antifungals.
- Prognosis poor in pediatric patients.

ICD Coding

- B46.8 - other zygomycoses

Epidemiology

- Ages 18 months to 80 years; male to female ratio of 11:1.
- Mean age 37 years.

Sites

- Mostly cause chronic infection in the skin and subcutaneous tissue.
- May cause infection in the stomach, small intestine, colon and liver.

Pathophysiology

- Infection is acquired by ingestion of infected food (e.g., people with pica) and using contaminated papers for cleaning the skin (e.g., toilet papers).
- Possibly due to ranitidine, which can decrease gastric acidity and allow fungal survival after gastric passing.
- Smoking can decrease mucosal WBC function and facilitate fungal infection by B. ranarum.

Etiology

- Basidiobolus ranarum

Clinical Features

- Abdominal pain and fever are most common presenting features.
- Other features include constipation, diarrhea, gastrointestinal bleeding, mucoid stool and rarely perforated appendicitis.

Diagnosis

- Based on characteristic histopathology findings of fungal hyphae (the Splendore-Hoeppli phenomenon) and culture of B. ranarum from the tissue specimen.

- The gold standard for definite diagnosis is culture.
- Macroscopically, colonies are yellowish gray in color with a waxy appearance and many radial folds.

Laboratory

- Eosinophilia and high ESR (erythrocyte sedimentation rate).
- Elevated levels of cytokines such as IL4, IL10, TNFα (TH2 type cytokines).

Radiology Description

- Colorectal mass is the most common finding, followed by hepatic mass or small bowel mass.
- Bowel wall thickening was noticed in 25% of the reported cases, whereas bowel perforation or abscess was less commonly seen.

Radiology Images

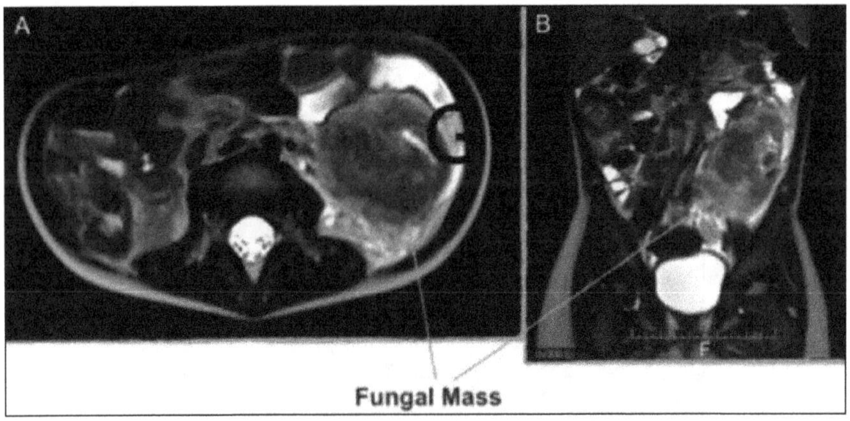

MRI before surgical intervention and treatment.

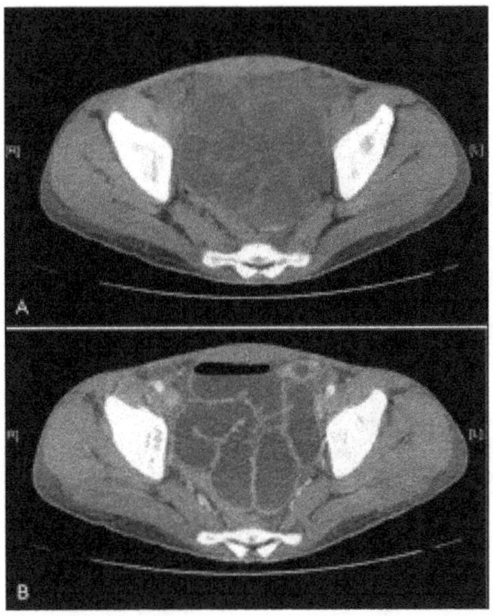

Generalized markedly thickened wall of the small bowel withedematous changes.

Poor Prognostic Factors

- Pediatric age group at presentation.
- Delayed treatment.

Treatment

- Combined surgery and antifungal treatment for a variable period of time (6 months to 2 years).
- Itraconazole, an antifungal agent is the most common drug used.

Gross Description

- Fungus involves the nonmucosal layers such as submucosa and subserosa of the GI tract, hence endoscopic biopsies, which are superficial and small, usually fail to detect the fungal hyphae.

Gross Images

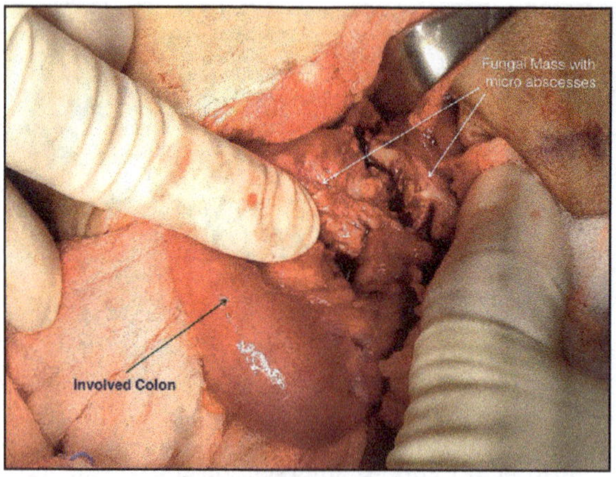

Edematous left colon.

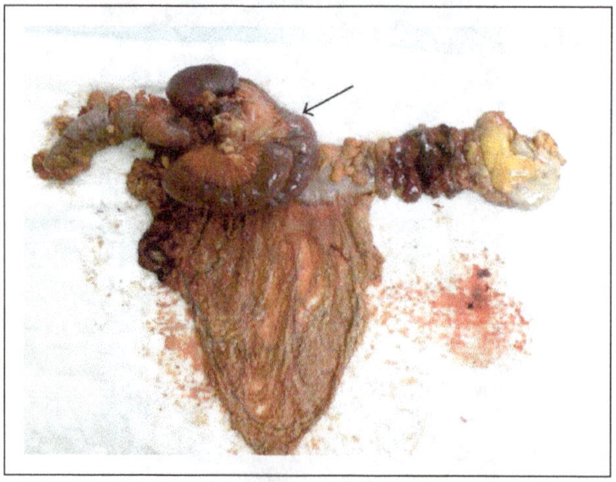

Adherent small bowel loop.

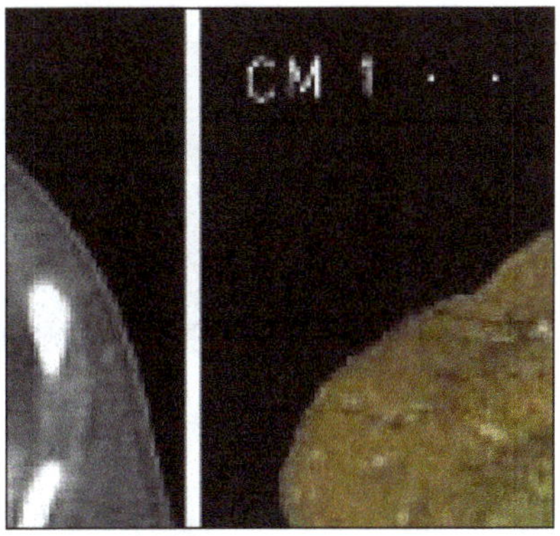

Postmortem liver.

Microscopic (Histologic) Description

- Marked infiltration of eosinophils.
- Mixed infiltration of PMN leukocytes and granulomatous inflammation.
- Thin wall and broad hyphae surrounded by eosinophilic material, which are easily seen by hematoxylin and eosin staining; however periodic acid-Schiff (PAS) and gomori methenamine silver (GMS) can intensify the fungal wall staining.
- Zygospores which are very similar to trophozoites of amoeba.

Microscopic (Histologic) Images

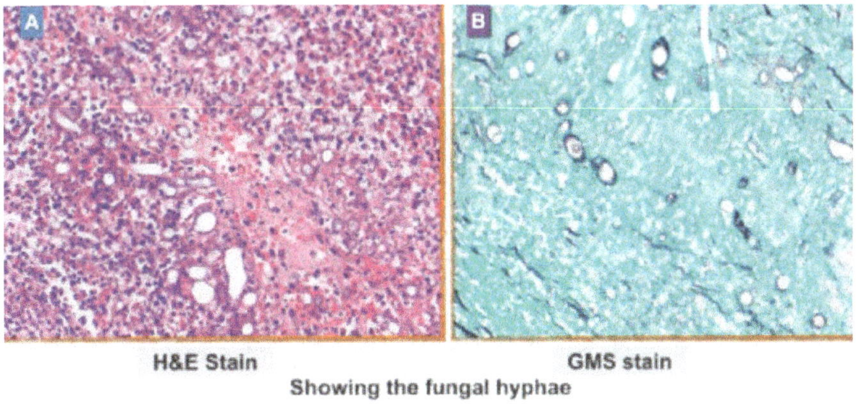

Staining of the tissue biopsy from left retrocolic mass.

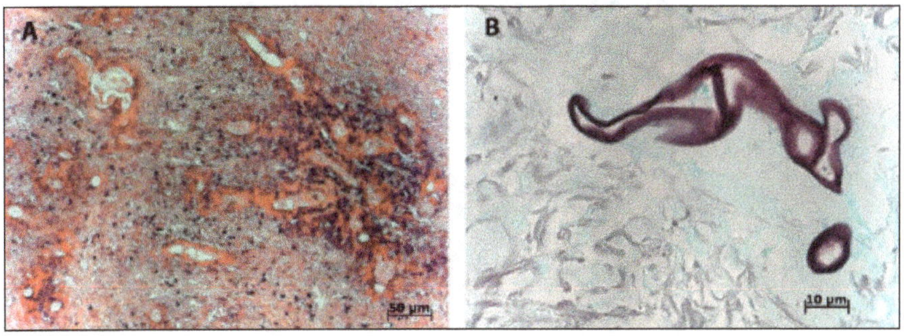

Histopathology of surgically resected abdominal mass.

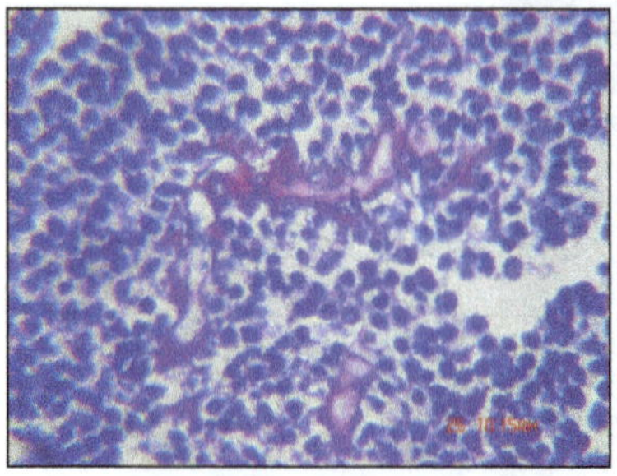

Broad hyphae with septation.

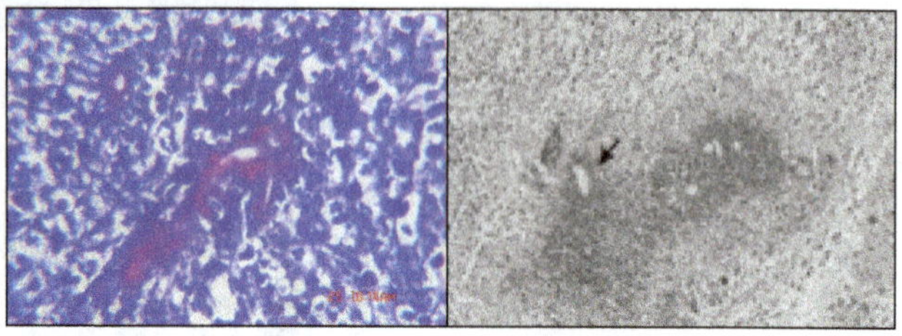

Splendore-Hoeppli phenomenon.

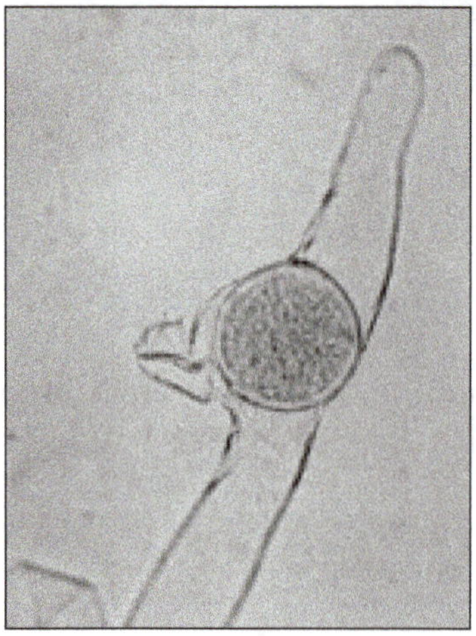

Zygospore.

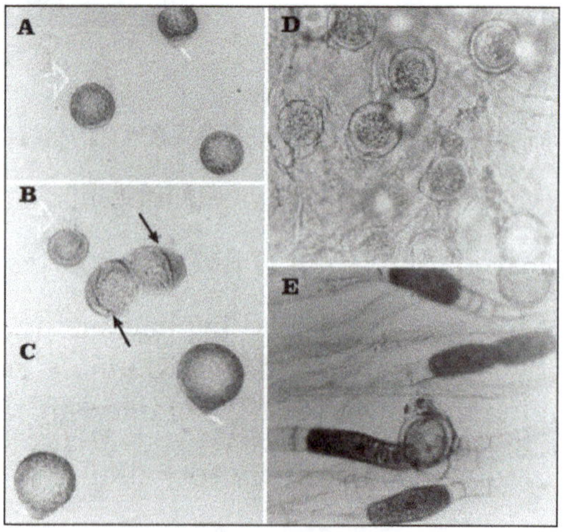

Spore forms.

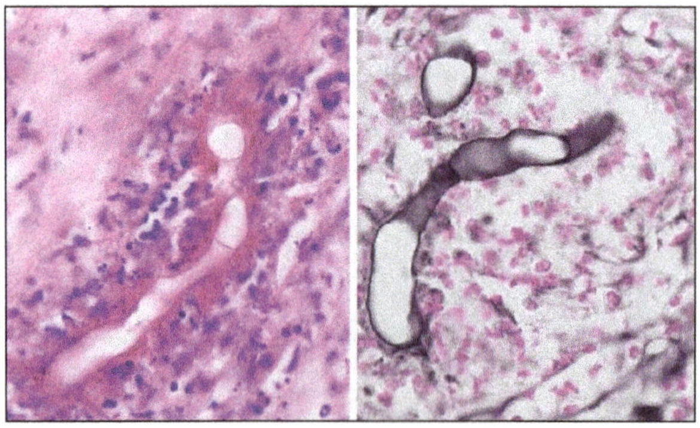

Liver biopsy.

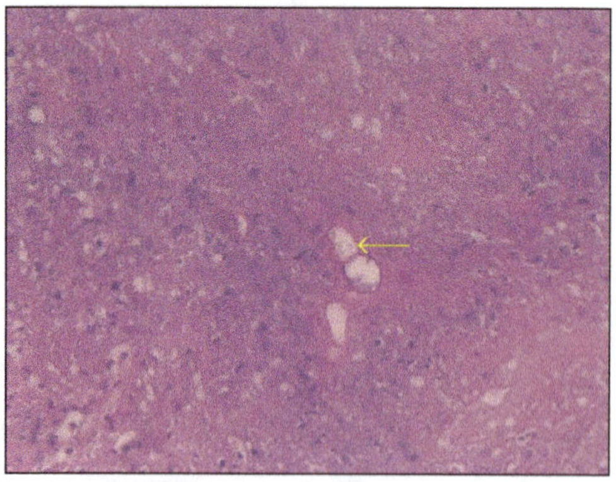

Periodic acid-Schiff stain.

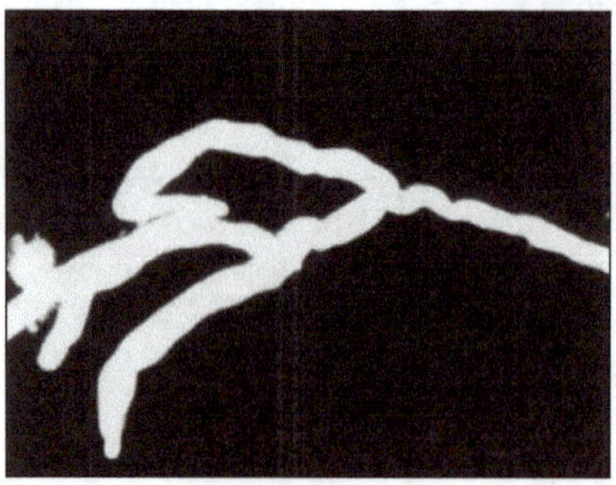

Various images.

Cytology Description

- Broad septate thin walled fungal hyphae along with eosinophils.

Positive Stains

- PAS, GMS

Differential Diagnosis

- Eosinophilic gastroenteritis: no fungal hyphae.
- Other granulomatous lesions: no broad septate fungal hyphae.

Rhinosporidiosis

Rhinosporidiosis is a rare, infectious, chronic granulomatous disease caused by Rhinosporidium seeberi, an endosporulating microorganism. It has recently been classified in the taxonomic group, mesomycetozoea, which is a group of microorganisms at the boundary between fish and fungi. The disease is most prevalent in warm, tropical climates, with over 90% of cases found in the Indian subcontinent. The nose and nasopharynx are most commonly involved at over 70% of reported cases, with ocular manifestations accounting for 15% of cases.

Clinical presentation of rhinosporidiosis depends on the location of the lesion and is typically found in mucosal membranes. The most common site of ocular lesions is the conjunctiva and lacrimal sac. Conjunctival rhinosporidiosis can be flat or pedunculated, depending on which area of the conjunctiva is involved and if there is space to grow. More uncommon sites include the lip, palate, maxillary antrum, uvula, epiglottis, larynx, trachea, bronchus, ear, vulva, penis, rectum, and scalp. In the rare occasion of a disseminated infection, limbs, trunks, viscera and brain can be involved, with brain involvement often leading to fatalities. According to Sinha et. al, there have been more reported male cases compared to females, but the difference is minimal (57% to 43%), with the majority of cases involving young adults. The younger age groups may be at risk due to the likelihood of young adults working outdoors or participating in outdoor activities.

Etiology

Rhinosporidiosis is an infection endemic to India, Sri Lanka, and Pakistan, Africa, and South America. It can also result from sporadic cases around the world. Rhinosporidiosis is caused by R. seeberi, which epidemiological evidence has found predominantly in stagnant water sources in tropical climates. Human-to-human transmission has not been identified, and therefore the disease is not considered contagious. Cases have also been reported in several species of farm, domestic, and wild animals such as dogs, cats, horses, cattle, ducks and swans.

The first reported case of rhinosporidiosis was in 1900 by Guillermo Seeber from Buenos Aires, who described a highly vascular nasal polyp. At that time the infectious agent was thought to be fungus and the classification of the species has been under debate for many years. In 1923, Asworth described the established the nomenclature, Rhinosporidium seeberi, after describing its life cycle.

Risk Factors

- Living near, or visiting a warm, tropical climate.
- Endemic regions such as India, Pakistan, Sri Lanka, African continent.
- Swimming or working near a stagnant water source (paddy workers, river-sand workers).
- Traumatized epithelium with Rhinosporidium exposure (by water or air).
- Inhalation of field dust contaminated by spores in feces of infected animals.

General Pathology

The pathology of Rhinosporidiosis stems from an infection from R. Seeberi, resulting in a highly vascular, often pedunculated soft tissue mass located in mucosal tissue such as nasopharynx, conjunctiva, and lacrimal sac.

Pathophysiology

Rhinosporidiosis is an infectious, highly vascular, polypoidal, soft tissue mass. It is caused by inoculation into a break of skin or from inhalation of Rhinosporidium seeberi. The reservoir for R. seeberi is stagnant water and soil. Despite being first identified in 1900, its classification has been under dispute due to its overlapping characteristics with fungi, fish, and amphibian pathogens. Human infection in the majority of reported cases is through contact of contaminated water with epithelial injury on the skin. The highest incidence of cases reported in river-sand workers.

Rhinosporidium seeberi is an infectious organism that is intractable to isolation and cannot be grown in artificial media. The microorganism can maintain its life cycle in tissue culture. Most reported cases show an association of rhinosporidiosis occurring in individuals in contact with stagnant, contaminated water. The infection occurs from inoculation of a site with R. seeberi in the form of endospores. These endospores develop into juvenile sporangia called trophocytes that do not contain any endospores. These trophocytes are 10-100 microns large, with a single layer of cells forming the cell wall. Trophocytes mature into intermediate sporangia which are larger, with thicker, bilamellar walls. Intermediate sporangia grow into mature sporangia, which are approximately 100-300 microns thick, filled with a large number of endospores, and surrounded by immune cells. Water or watery substance stimulates the endospores to be released from the sporangia perpetuating the infection and life cycle. After initial infection with R. seeberi, replication occurs rapidly in the mucosa at the site of infection with hyperplasia of host tissue and recruitment of local immune response to develop the lesion. This immune response to the infection leads to the formation of a granuloma and further develops into a multilobulated mass at the site of infection.

Primary Prevention

Primary prevention is to avoid swimming in stagnant water, particularly in warm, tropical climates, or endemic regions.

Diagnosis

Histopathology is the definitive way to confirm a diagnosis of Rhinosporidiosis. On histopathology, visible trophocytes and sporangia will be in different stages of development with surrounding infiltration of inflammatory cells and hyperplasia of the mucosal tissue.

History

Patients presenting with rhinosporidiosis may often have a history of swimming in stagnant water, have recent travel or residence in endemic areas, work near rivers or are river-sand workers.

Physical Examination

Rhinosporidiosis occurs when the endospores of R. seeberi infect the mucosa through a traumatized epithelium, leading to hyperplasia and growth of a soft lesion on the site of infection. It can present in various locations in the body, but predominantly arise in the nasal passage, eyes and oropharynx. Rhinosporidium polyps appear as a soft tissue lesion that is granular, fleshy, and red in color with multiple yellowish to white pin head sized dots that indicate underlying mature sporangia. Depending on the location, the lesion can present as pedunculated or flat.

In Sinha et al, nasopharyngeal lesions are described as often being multi-lobed and less vascular. Patients often complain of epistaxis, nasal obstruction, rhinorrhea, anosmia. Conjunctival rhinosporidiosis presents with a similarly fleshy lesion, which can be pedunculated if formed in palpebral conjunctiva or flat if formed in the bulbar conjunctiva. Bulbar conjunctival lesions are typically sessile and flat as the lids over the conjunctiva exert a flattening force. Patients present with symptoms of watery eyes, conjunctivitis, photophobia. If the lacrimal sac is involved, bloody tears may be present.

Signs

- Pedunculated, or flat sessile soft tissue growth.
- Fleshy appearance.
- Pinpoint white or yellow spots.
- Highly vascular and friable with free bleeding.
- Proptosis.

Symptoms

- Watering of eyes (ocular lesion).
- Conjunctivitis (ocular lesion).
- Bloody Tears (ocular lesion).
- Photophobia (ocular lesion).

- Itching (ocular and nasopharynx lesion).
- Difficulty breathing (nasopharynx lesion).
- Rhinorrhea (nasopharynx lesion).
- Anosmia (nasopharynx lesion).
- Epistaxis (nasopharynx lesion).
- Difficulty swallowing (oropharynx lesion).

Diagnostic Procedures

Definitive diagnosis of rhinosporidiosis depends on histological examination with immunohistochemistry. This often requires excisional biopsy, scraping of superficial lesions or fine needle aspiration. The histopathological sections will show sporangia in multiple stages of maturation enclosed within a thin wall. The sporangia can range from 50-1000 µm in diameter with endospores inside that are approximately 5-10 µm. The overlying and surrounding tissue has rapid growth with the infection with hyperplasia of the tissue and loose fibrovascular stroma. Immune reactions to the infection also results in infiltration with lymphocytes, macrophages, plasma cells and PMNs. Rupture of the sporangia can result in a giant cell reaction. Despite having overlapping characteristics with fungi, R. seeberi lacks the Splendore-Hoeppli reaction, which is characterized by an eosinophilic infiltration. A key characteristic of rhinosporidiosis is that the infected site is almost completely devoid of eosinophils.

Multiple stains can assist in the diagnosis of rhinosporidiosis. The sporangia and endospores stain positively to various special stains such as Mucicarmine, Gomori's methenamine-silver, PAS, etc. Nasopharyngeal polyps are the most commonly infected sites, and identification of endospores is often difficult when compared to epithelial cells of the respiratory sites. Periodic Acid Schiff (PAS) staining is helpful to use as endospores are PAS positive, but PAS negative in epithelial cells. Mucicarmine stain can be helpful in distinguishing R. Seeberi (stains positively) from Coccidiodes immitis (does not stain positively). Furthermore, cytologically, coccidiomycotic lesions can often look similar to rhinosporidial lesions as both are represented by large, thick- sporangia containing small endospores. However, using H and E staining can show that R. seeberi endospores are larger and more numerous than C. immitis.

Differential Diagnosis

- Pyogenic granuloma,
- Squamous or conjunctival papilloma,
- Hemangioma,
- Arteriovenous malformation,
- Chronic infection,
- Oncocytoma,

- Sebaceous adenoma,
- Squamous carcinoma,
- Foreign body,
- Conjunctival cyst,
- Inflamed pinguecula.

Management

Rhinosporidiosis infection is treated primarily with surgical intervention. Medical management has rarely been reported as adjunct treatment to surgery.

General Treatment

Th first line treatment of rhinosporidiosis is surgical, and the method utilized is dictated by the location of the lesion. In the majority of cases, total surgical excision is completed using cautery. Electrocautery minimizes the bleeding from the highly vascular structure and limits the release of endospores into the nearby mucosa. This may decrease the chance of recurrence.

Medical treatment with Dapsone and Amphotericin B is possible, but not well studied. Efficacy of these drugs are controversial, but may be used in disseminated disease. Dapsone has been used in a few case reports but always as an adjunct to surgical treatment. As R. seeberi cannot be grown in vitro, drug sensitivities are currently unknown.

Medical Therapy

Medical management of rhinosporidiosis has not been strongly advised in reported cases. Currently, dapsone is an adjuvant drug to surgery.

Surgery

Total excision of the polyp or conjunctiva is recommended, and electrocautery is most commonly utilized as it restricts free bleeding. If there is lacrimal sac involvement, a dacryocystectomy is typically done. The procedure should remove the entirety of the entire sac, and post-operative Dapsone therapy is usually recommended. In a retrospective case series from India, 65% of all patients with lacrimal sac involvement had localized disease. During removal of the polyp, spillage of the endospores into the surrounding mucosa may occur which can be contained by electrocautery.

Complications

Complications of rhinosporidiosis are relatively rare. Disseminated infection may occur leading to osteolytic bone lesions which may be difficult to distinguish from relapse or reinfection in endemic regions. Disseminated infection of the limbs can lead to bone destruction or infection of the brain and other sites of the body. It is difficult to treat and can lead to increased morbidity. In addition, local secondary bacterial infections are significant complications that can lead to morbidity as well. Recurrence rates of ocular rhinosporidiosis is lower than that of nasopharyngeal rhinosporidiosis.

Prognosis

Despite the rare case of recurrence, regeneration or dissemination, the prognosis is generally very favorable. It typically follows a benign, prolonged course without treatment with limited morbidity. Morbidity is typically associated when there is a secondary infection or dissemination occurs.

Sporotrichosis

Sporotrichosis is a rare type of fungal infection that can occur in both humans and animals. Also nicknamed "rose handler's disease," the fungus can be found in certain plants and their surrounding soil. Sporotrichosis mostly affects people who work with these products, such as:

- Farmers.
- Florists.
- Gardeners.
- Those who work at plant nurseries.
- Those who handle bales of hay.
- Carpenters.

While rare and usually not life-threatening, this type of fungal infection can lead to serious complications.

Pictures of Sporotrichosis

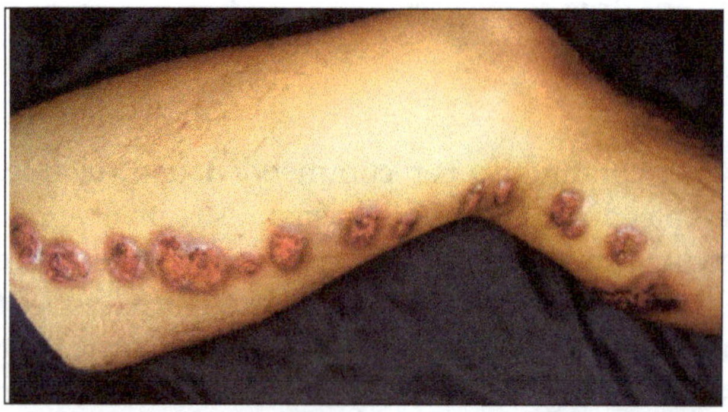

Lesions and nodules appear along the lymph node drainage lines when people become infected with sporotrichosis.

Symptoms of Sporotrichosis

The symptoms of sporotrichosis often start off mild within the first several weeks of exposure. You'll experience a small bump that can be red, pink, or purple. This bump appears at the site of exposure, usually on your arm or hand, and may or may not be painful to the touch. It can take 1 to 12 weeks before sporotrichosis shows any symptoms.

As the infection progresses, the bump can turn into an ulcer. You may have a severe rash surrounding the affected area, as well as new bumps that surface. Sometimes the rash can affect your eyes, and even cause conjunctivitis (commonly called pink eye).

Causes of Sporotrichosis

Sporotrichosis is caused by the *Sporothrix* fungus. This type of fungus is prevalent in all parts of the world, but it may be more common in Central and South America. According to the U.S. Centers for Disease Control and Prevention (CDC), the fungus may be found in rose bushes, hay, and moss. If you handle any of these plants or their surrounding soil on a regular basis, you could be at risk for exposure to the fungus. Still, exposure doesn't automatically mean you'll develop a fungal infection.

Cutaneous Sporotrichosis

Having an open cut or wound on your skin can put you at risk for cutaneous sporotrichosis. This means that the fungus enters your skin. Some people become infected after getting cut by a plant containing the fungus — this is why rose thorns are noteworthy culprits of possible sporotrichosis.

Pulmonary Sporotrichosis

Rarely, the fungus can enter your lungs after you breathe in spores from the air. This subtype is called pulmonary sporotrichosis. It may cause breathing difficulties, chest pain, cough, fever, fatigue, and unintentional weight loss.

Sporotrichosis can also be spread to humans from infected animals (especially cats) through scratches and bites. However, it isn't spread between people. According to BMJ Case Reports, the highest rates of infection tend to occur in people between the ages of 16 and 30.

Ways of Diagnosing Sporotrichosis

To properly diagnose sporotrichosis, you'll need to see your doctor for testing. They will take a skin sample called a biopsy, and then submit it to the lab. If your doctor suspects pulmonary sporotrichosis, they may order a blood test. Sometimes blood tests can also help diagnose severe forms of cutaneous sporotrichosis.

Getting the right treatment depends on the results of these tests.

Home Treatments for Sporotrichosis

Fungal infections like sporotrichosis depend on medical treatments to get rid of the fungus from the body. However, some home treatments can help decrease the spread of the infection. For skin infections, you can make sure that the wound is kept clean and bandaged. This can help prevent any rashes from getting worse. You'll also want to make sure you avoid scratching the area.

Treatments for Sporotrichosis

Skin infections from this type of fungus are treated with antifungals, such as oral itraconazole

(Sporanox) and supersaturated potassium iodide. These are taken for several months until the infection has fully cleared up.

Severe sporotrichosis may need intravenous (IV) treatments, such as amphotericin B. According to the CDC, you may need to take itraconazole for up to one year after your IV treatments are complete. This helps ensure that the fungus is completely out of your body.

If the infection originated in your lungs, you may need to have surgery. The process involves cutting out infected lung tissue.

Complications of Sporotrichosis

Most cases of sporotrichosis aren't deadly. However, if you don't treat the infection, you could have the bumps and sores for many years. Some cases can become permanent.

Left untreated, this type of infection can develop into disseminated sporotrichosis. With this condition, the fungal infection spreads to other body parts. Examples include your bones or your central nervous system. You might experience:

- Joint pain.
- Severe headaches.
- Confusion.
- Seizures.

A weakened immune system can put you at risk for this type of sporotrichosis, especially if you have HIV.

Hyalohyphomycosis

Hyalohyphomycosis is infection caused by nonpigmented fungi (other than the genera *Aspergillus* or *Penicillium* or the class Zygomycetes) that in tissue form hyphal elements with hyaline or clear walls. Examples of genera causing hyalohyphomycosis in people and other animals include *Acremonium, Fusarium, Geotrichum, Paecilomyces, Pseudallescheria, Sagenomella, Phialosimplex, Geosmithia, Geomyces,* and *Scedosporium*. Hyalohyphomycosis is far less common than phaeohyphomycosis.

Clinical Findings

Lesions range from local cutaneous, subcutaneous, corneal, or nasal mucosal disease to disseminated disease involving the lungs and multiple other organ systems. Disseminated and corneal forms have been reported most commonly. Animals presenting with cutaneous lesions should be evaluated for systemic disease. Animals being treated with immunosuppressive drugs for immune-mediated disease may develop cutaneous hyalohyphomycosis and not have lesions at other sites, whereas immunocompetent animals that develop hyalohyphomycosis most often do have disseminated disease, or at least disease that is not confined to the skin.

Diagnosis

The several causative fungi cannot be identified by their histologic features in tissues; culture isolation and/or PCR are required.

Treatment

Surgical removal with or without azole antifungal therapy is the treatment of choice for local disease. Disseminated disease typically carries a grave prognosis. Treatment with newer azole antifungals and/or amphotericin B lipid complex may be attempted and is most likely to be effective if immunosuppressive drugs can be tapered.

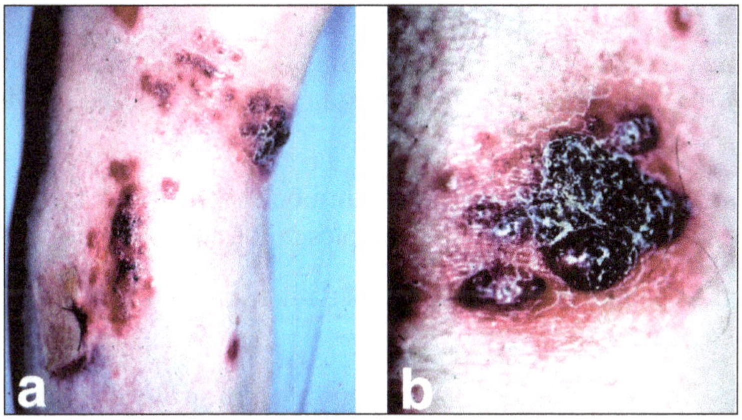

Talaromyces Marneffei

Talaromyces marneffei, formerly called *Penicillium marneffei*, was identified in 1956. The organism is endemic to southeast Asia where it is an important cause of opportunistic infections in those with HIV/AIDS-related immunodeficiency. Incidence of *T. marneffei* infections has increased due to a rise in HIV infection rates in the region.

When it was classified as a *Penicillium*, it was the only known thermally dimorphic species of that genus that caused a lethal systemic infection (talaromycosis), with fever and anaemia similar to disseminated cryptococcosis. This contrasted with related *Penicillium* species that are usually regarded as unimportant in terms of causing human disease.

Epidemiology

There is a high incidence of talaromycosis in AIDS patients in SE Asia; 10% of patients in Hong Kong get talaromycosis as an AIDS-related illness. Cases of *T. marneffei* human infections (talaromycosis) have also been reported in HIV-positive patients in Australia, Europe, Japan, the UK and the U.S. All the patients, except one, had visited Southeast Asia previously. The disease is considered an AIDS-defining illness.

Discovered in bamboo rats (*Rhizomys*) in Vietnam, it is associated with these rats and the tropical

Southeast Asia area. *Talaromyces marneffei* is endemic in Myanmar (Burma), Cambodia, Southern China, Indonesia, Laos, Malaysia, Thailand and Vietnam.

Although both the immunocompetent and the immunocompromised can be infected, it is extremely rare to find systemic infections in HIV-negative patients. The incidence of *T. marneffei* is increasing as HIV spreads throughout Asia. An increase in global travel and migration means it will be of increased importance as an infection in AIDS sufferers.

Talaromyces marneffei has been found in bamboo rat faeces, liver, lungs and spleen. It has been suggested that these animals serve as a reservoir for the fungus. It is not clear whether the rats are affected by *T. marneffei* or are merely asymptomatic carriers of the disease.

One study of 550 AIDS patients showed that the incidence was higher during the rainy season, which is when the rats breed. But this season also has conditions that are more favorable for production of fungal spores (conidia), which can become airborne and be inhaled by susceptible individuals.

Another study could not establish contact with bamboo rats as a risk factor, but exposure to the soil was the critical risk factor. However, soil samples failed to yield much of the fungus.

It is not known whether people get the disease by eating infected rats, or by inhaling fungi from their faeces.

One HIV-positive physician is known to have been infected while attending a course on tropical microbiology. He did not handle the organism, though students in the same laboratory did. It is presumed he contracted the infection by inhaling aerosol containing *T. marneffei* conidia. This shows that airborne infections are possible.

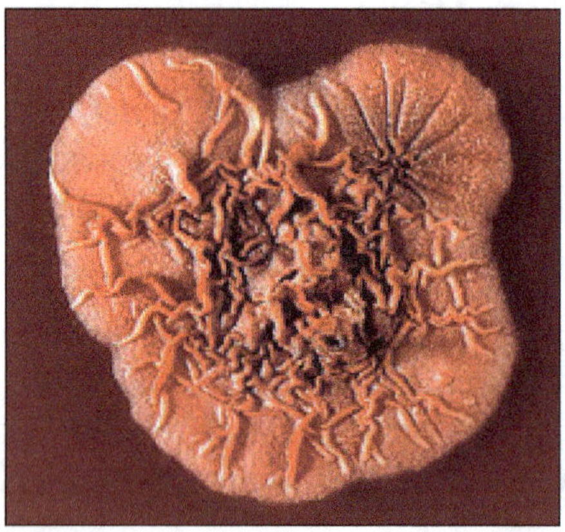

The surface of a *Talaromyces* (formerly *Penicillium*) *marneffei* colony.

Clinical Presentation

Patients commonly present with symptoms and signs of infection of the reticuloendothelial system, including generalized lymphadenopathy, hepatomegaly, and splenomegaly. The respiratory system is commonly involved as well; cough, fever, dyspnea, and chest pain may be present, reflecting the probable inhalational route of acquisition. Approximately one-third of patients may also exhibit gastrointestinal symptoms, such as diarrhea.

Laboratory Diagnosis

The fact that *Talaromyces marneffei* is thermally dimorphic is a relevant clue when trying to identify it. However, it should be kept in mind that other human-pathogenic fungi are thermally dimorphic as well. Cultures should be done from bone marrow, skin, blood and sputum samples.

Plating samples out onto two Sabouraud agar plates, then incubating one at 30 °C and the other at 37 °C, should result in two different morphologies. A mold-form will grow at 30 °C, and a yeast-form at 37 °C.

Mycelial colonies will be visible on the 30 °C plate after two days. Growth is initially fluffy and white and eventually turns green and granular after sporulation has occurred. A soluble red pigment is produced, which diffuses into the agar, causing the reverse side of the plate to appear red or pink. The periphery of the mold may appear orange-coloured, and radial sulcate folds will develop.

Under the microscope, the mold phase will look like a typical *Penicillium*, with hyaline, septate and branched hyphae; the conidiophores are located both laterally and terminally. Each conidiophore gives rise to three to five phialides, where chains of lemon-shaped conidia are formed.

On the 37 °C plate, the colonies grow as yeasts. These colonies can be cerebriform, convoluted, or smooth. There is a decreased production in pigment, the colonies appearing cream/light-tan/light-pink in colour. Microscopically, sausage-shaped cells are mixed with hyphae-like structures. As the culture ages, segments begin to form. The cells divide by binary fission, rather than budding. The cells are not yeast cells, but rather arthroconidia. Culturing isn't the only method of diagnosis. A skin scraping can be prepared, and stained with Wright's stain. Many intracellular and extracellular yeast cells with crosswalls are suggestive of *T. marneffei* infection. Smears from bone marrow aspirates may also be taken; this is regarded as the most sensitive method. These samples can be stained with the Giemsa stain. Histological examination can also be done on skin, bone marrow or lymph nodes.

The patient's history also is a diagnostic help. If they have traveled to Southeast Asia and are HIV-positive, then there is an increased risk of them having talaromycosis.

Antigen testing of urine and serum, and PCR amplification of specific nucleotide sequences have been tried, with high sensitivity and specificity. Rapid identification of talaromycosis is sought, as prompt treatment is critical. Treatment should be provided as soon as talaromycosis is suspected.

Treatment

Treatment of talaromycosis depends on the degree of immunosuppression and organ involvement, but most isolates of Talaromyces marneffei display low MIC's to amphotericin B as well as itraconazole, posaconazole and voriconazole.

Phaeohyphomycosis

Phaeohyphomycosis refers to a group of mycoses (fungal infections) that are dematiaceous, which means they are pigmented. The pigment is due to their ability to deposit melanin in their cell walls.

Histology of Phaeohyphomycosis

Scanning power view of phaeohyphomycosis shows a deeply extending granulomatous pattern which may show areas of necrosis. Centrally an abscess or cystic nodule may form. Frequently a foreign body such as a wood splinter can be seen. The epidermis commonly shows pseudoepitheliomatous hyperplasia. The inflammatory infiltrate is comprised of histiocytes with multinucleated giant cells, and numerous neutrophils. At high power branching septate pigmented fungal hyphae can be seen.

Phaeohyphomycosis Pathology

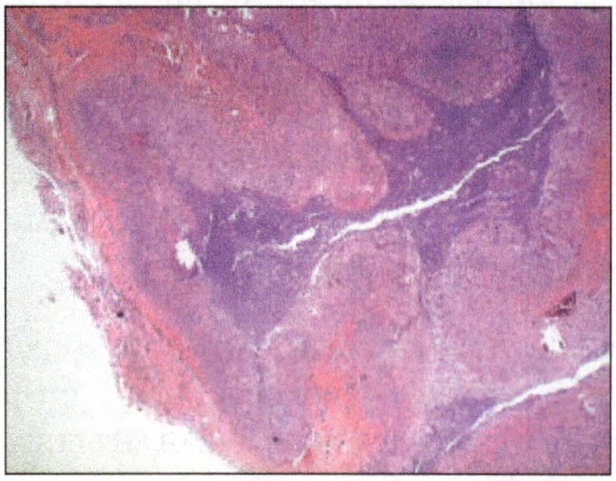

Phaeohyphomycosis pathology.

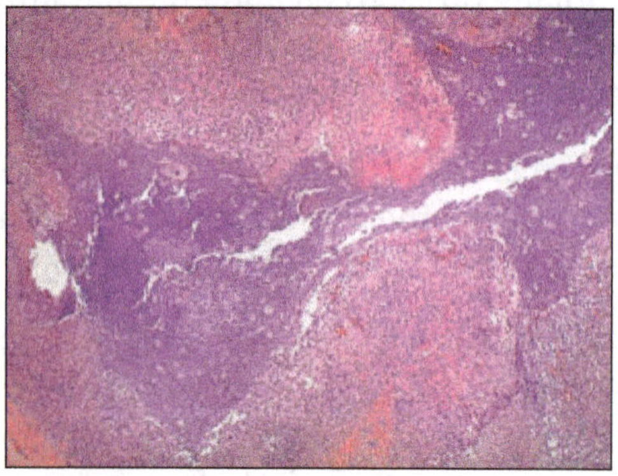

Phaeohyphomycosis pathology.

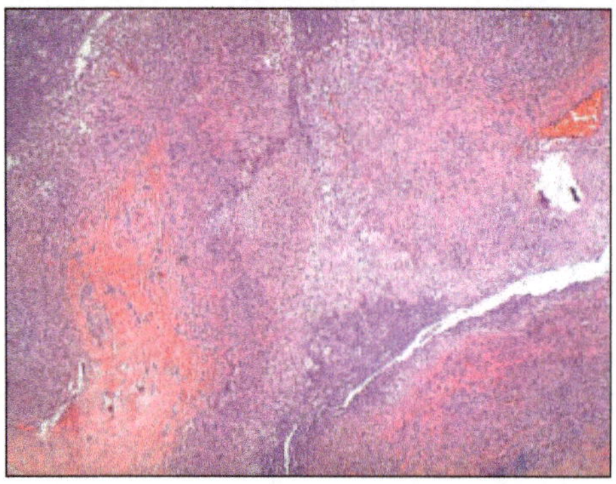

Phaeohyphomycosis pathology.

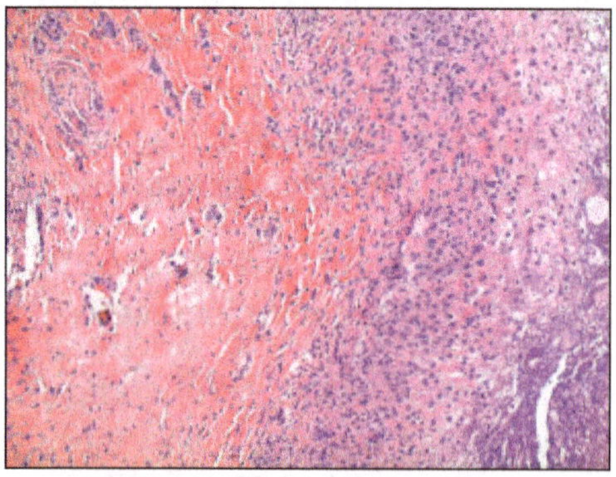

Phaeohyphomycosis pathology.

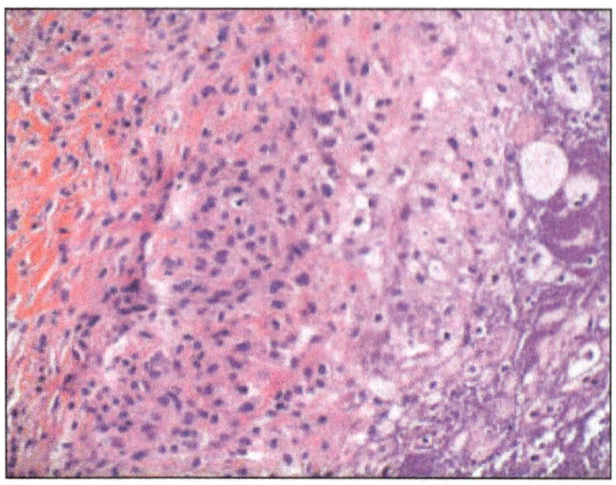

Phaeohyphomycosis pathology.

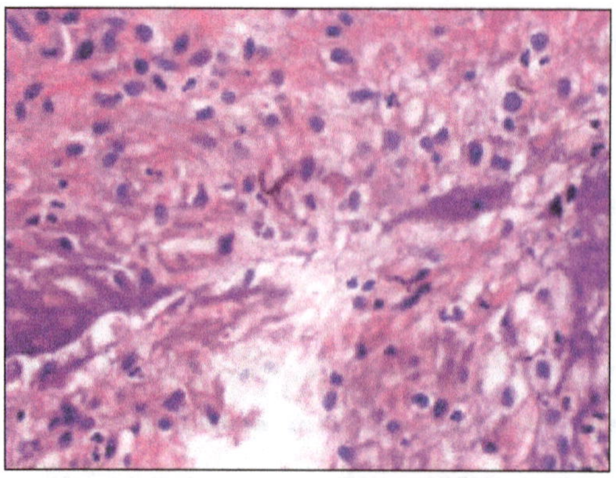

Phaeohyphomycosis pathology.

Special Stains in Phaeohyphomycosis

PAS or Grocott methenamine silver stains can be used to enhance visualisation of the fungal hyphae.

Phaeohyphomycosis Pathology, PAS Stain

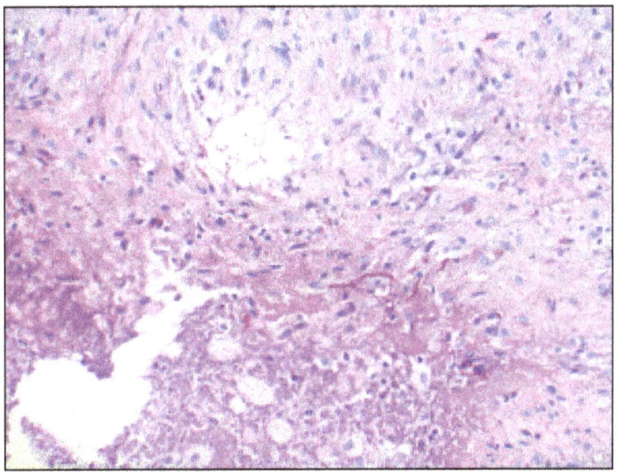

Phaeohyphomycosis pathology.

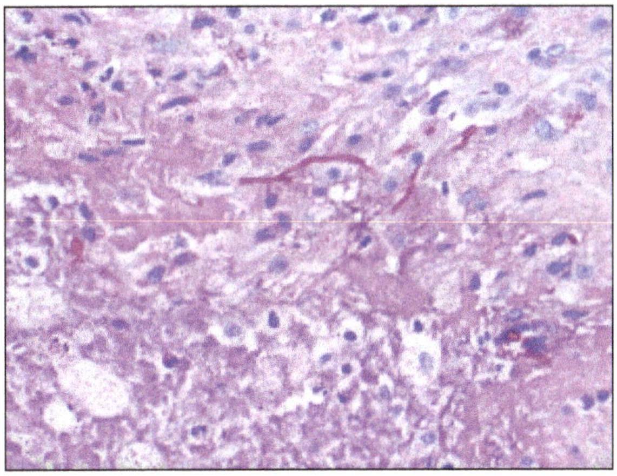

Phaeohyphomycosis pathology, PAS stain.

Differential Diagnosis of Phaeohyphomycosis

Chromomycosis: This pigmented fungal infection demonstrates formation of rounded sclerotic or septate bodies/muriform cells.

Invasive Malassezia Infections

Malassezia (formerly known as *Pityrosporum*) species are members of human cutaneous commensal flora, which are associated with a wide spectrum of clinical manifestations from benign skin conditions, such as tinea versicolor and folliculitis, to fungemia in the immunocompromised host.

The epidemiology, clinical manifestations, diagnosis, and treatment of invasive *Malassezia* infections will be discussed here. The clinical manifestations, diagnosis, and treatment of tinea versicolor and *Malassezia* folliculitis are discussed elsewhere.

Mycology

Malassezia are lipophilic yeasts that are constituents of the normal human skin flora. Studies have revealed that many *Malassezia* species produce biofilm, which is used during attachment to host and other surfaces. These organisms have been classified into at least 17 species, including *M. furfur*, *M. pachydermatis*, *M. sympodialis*, *M. slooffiae*, *M. obtusa*, *M. globosa*, and *M. restricta*, based upon polymerase chain reaction and restriction endonuclease analysis. A study has reported reliable species identification by matrix-assisted laser desorption/ionization time-of-flight (MALDI-TOF) mass spectrometry following the development of a MALDI-TOF database. In another study evaluating 392 clinical isolates (identified by sequencing) from patients with *Malassezia* folliculitis and pityriasis versicolor, 68 percent were *M. furfur* and 19 percent were *M. globosa*.

Epidemiology

Malassezia species mainly colonize the skin and occasionally the respiratory tract. The organisms appear to become part of the normal skin flora by three to six months of age. *M. furfur* was recovered from the skin in 32 to 64 percent of neonates in neonatal intensive care units in two separate series. In one study, duration of stay in the unit and gestational age were factors favoring skin colonization.

Colonization of the skin with *Malassezia* and subsequent extension to central venous catheters appears more common in neonates than adults. Studies using scanning electron microscopy have demonstrated that some *Malassezia* spp produce significant biofilms. *M. furfur* was recovered from the lumen in 32 percent of percutaneous central venous catheters in a neonatal intensive care unit in one series but not from the insertion sites in 928 adults receiving total parenteral nutrition.

Keratomycosis

Fungal keratitis is a serious ocular infection with potentially catastrophic visual results. Caused by any of the many species of fungi capable of colonizing human tissue, its occurs worldwide and its incidence is increasing in frequency.

Etiology

The list covers many fungi including but not limited to yeasts of Candida spp., filamentous with septae such as Aspergillus spp., Fusarium spp., Cladosporium,spp., Curvularia, and non septated such as Rhizopus. Bear in mind that any agent capable of infecting humans is a potential infectious agent, especially if the host has a debilitating disease.

Risk Factors

Risk factors include trauma, ocular surface disease, and topical steroid use. Risks and type of fungi also might vary by geographic location and climate. In warmer climates the rule is that the most common organisms are filamentous fungi, like Fusarium spp and Aspergillus spp. with a strong relationship to trauma. Reports from Brazil show the most common isolates in descending order were Fusarium spp in 67%, Aspergillus spp in 10.5%, and Candida spp in 10%. About 40% of the infections were related to trauma.

In the northern USA, corneal infection by fungus was, until recently, more common in debilitated or immunocompromised patients and the causative organism being a yeast, such as Candida albicans. Filamentous fungi in these latitudes were then rarely reported. A few years ago a breakout of Fusarium keratitis associated with a type of contact lens solution displaced yeasts as the most common fungal corneal infection in some areas. This trend persists in the most recent epidemiological reports. Still they are, in most cases, related to contact lens use. It should be noted that the incidence of contact lens-related fungal keratitis was increasing before the Fusarium outbreak.

This new distribution means that we no longer can rely on the geographical distribution only to initiate empirical treatment. Broad-spectrum treatment should be administerd once there is a strong probability of a mycotic infection.

General Pathology

Even though fungi can be classified as a kingdom due to their complexity and unique characteristics, a simple practical classification for ocular infection is used. Under this method, morphology and type of reproductive method define the type of fungi. They are classified for our purpose as yeast, filamentous septated pigmented and non-pigmented and filamentous without septae. Fungi are present worldwide and can be part of the ocular flora. They are eukaryotic with a defined nucleus surrounded by a membrane. They can be either saprophytic, free organisms that subsist on decaying organic matter or pathologic and require a living host for perpetuation.

The American Academy of Ophthalmology's Pathology Atlas contains virtual microscopy images of tissue samples with the following:

- Aspergillus Keratitis
- Fungal Keratitis

Pathophysiology

The infection probably starts when the epithelial integrity is broken either due to trauma or ocular surface disease and the organism gains access into the tissue and proliferates. Proteolytic enzymes, fungal antigens and toxins are liberated into the cornea with the resulting necrosis and damage to its architecture thus compromising the eye integrity and function.

Primary Prevention

Wearing safety glasses while gardening will diminish the risk of ocular trauma. Also, general hygiene, proper contact lens care, and avoidance of nonessential steroid use should diminish the probability of mycotic infection.

Diagnosis

A high degree of suspicion from the physician accounts for early diagnosis and treatment, which are paramount for a successful resolution of the fungal keratitis. Corneal ulcers unresponsive to broad-spectrum antibiotics, the presence of satellite lesions, and scanty secretions in a large ulcer are some signs that should raise flags to the attending professional about the possibility of a mycotic agent.

History

Blurred vision, redness, tearing, photophobia, pain, foreign body sensations, secretions related to trauma, ocular surface disease and topical steroid use are all important characteristics to ascertain in the history.

Physical Examination

After establishing the patient's general condition, the examiner should look for evidence of ocular surface disease and determine the amount and type of secretions and lid swelling. The upper eyelid should be everted to exclude a retained foreign body. The examiner should measure the size and depth of the lesion as well as the presence of satellite lesions. The intraocular pressure should also be ascertained. Anterior chamber reaction and evidence of hypopyon should also be recorded. Vitreous reaction if present may suggest intraocular spread of the disease.

Signs

With filamentary fungi, the corneal lesions have a white/gray infiltrate with feathery borders. There might be satellite lesions with a hypopyon and conjunctival injection as well as purulent secretions. Ulcers caused by yeast are plaque-like and slightly more defined, similar to bacterial keratitis.

Symptoms

Symptoms are similar to any corneal infection including blurred vision, redness, tearing, photophobia, pain, foreign body sensation and secretions. In some cases the lesion are rather indolent which help to delay the diagnosis and hence delay the treatment. Suspicion should be high in cases of trauma with vegetable matter.

Clinical Diagnosis

Under the slit lamp, early on the lesion might look like an unhealed corneal abrasion with scanty infiltrates and no secretions. With time however, the ulcer develops thicker infiltrates and fuzzy margins. The presence of satellite lesions strongly suggests a fungal infection. Redness and periocular edema are also common. This combined with a history of trauma, especially with vegetable matter, ocular surface disease or chronic use of topical steroids should alert the practitioner to the possibility of a mycotic etiology.

Diagnostic Procedures

Corneal scrapings are taken from deep within the lesion with a surgical blade or sterile spatula. To perform a corneal biopsy, a dermatological 2mm punch can be used.

Laboratory Test

For a definitive diagnosis, scrapings taken from deep within the lesion should be made and inoculated in Sabouraud agar. The shortcoming is that it can take up to 3 weeks to grow and identify the organism. For a faster result, smears with special stains such as Gomori, PAS, acridine orange, calcofluor white or KOH should be performed. The drawback is that not all laboratories have these stains available, so, again we might need to rely on the patient's evolution and the physician's clinical acumen. If all labs and cultures are negative, corneal biopsy should be considered to obtain a specimen.

Differential Diagnosis

Fungal infections can mimic any microbial keratitis secondary to other causes: Bacteria, which is the most common cause of corneal infections; Acanthamoeba, related to swimming with contact lenses and or the use of tap water in their cleaning; or herpes simplex or herpes zoster for which recurrences are frequent. Other conditions such as a retained foreign body, sterile infiltrates, marginal ulcers due to Staphylococcal hypersensitivity or chronic epithelial defect should also be ruled out. Again, a high index of suspicion is important in the diagnosis of fungal keratitis. In recent times, there are a large number of cases being reported secondary to Pythium keratitis, which is a close mimicker of fungal keratitis. The features mimicking fungal keratitis are stromal infiltrate, ring ulceration, hypopyon, endothelial exudates and corneal perforation. The classical hallmark feature of Pythium keratitis include reticular dot like infiltrate, tentacular projections, early limbal and peripheral furrowing.

Management

In general, management consists of medical therapy with the use of topical and/or systemic anti-fungal medications alone or in combination with surgical treatment.

General Treatment

Topical antifungals, either commercially available or compounded from systemic preparation into eye-drops are the backbone for the management of fungal keratitis. In resistant cases, the addition of systemic antifungal have shown effectiveness. If those treatments fail, then conjunctival flaps , lamellar or penetrating keratoplasty might be needed.

Medical Therapy

Fungal ulcers are inherently difficult to treat. The diagnosis is often delayed and medications available for ocular therapy are limited and are deficient in their ability to penetrate deep into the cornea. The mainstay of treatment is the use of antifungal drops but only a polyene, natamycin 5%, is FDA approved and commercially available for topical ocular use. Also, due to the rarity of the diagnosis it is sometimes available only as a special order. Furthermore, the complexity of the disease and possible visually devastating outcomes require a rather aggressive approach to its treatment. Hence, many other antimycotics are used to fight this infection. These compounded eye drops are made by diluting the intravenous medication into concentrations that provide enough medication to eradicate the organism while being tolerated by the eye.

Prior to the development of natamycin the most commonly used antifungal was amphotericin b, a polyene, in a 0.15% dilution in sterile water (one 50mg vial of amphotericin b diluted in 30cc sterile water gives a 0.166% dilution). It is still used today alone and in combination with natamycin with relatively good results. Since they both are readily available, they are both a good choice as initial therapy.

Voriconazole, a triazole antifungal agent derived from fluconazole, can be used either topically at 1% dilution, orally at 400 mg twice a day and even has being injected in the corneal stroma around the fungal lesion (50 micrograms/0.1 ml).

Oral posaconazole, a new generation triazole, has been successful eradicating deep infections of resistant Fusarium Subconjuctival antifungals are not generally used because the produce severe pain and some might even induce tissue necrosis.

Other antifungals available include the azoles like miconazole, clotrimazole ketoconazole, posaconazole, and fluconazole and the echinocandin antifungal agents caspofungin, and micafungin. The echinocandins are not active against Fusarium.

Medical Follow Up

All corneal infections should be followed daily until there is a marked improvement. Since fungal infections run a protracted course, their follow up is longer and after a few days the interval between evaluations increases according to its progress. Complete healing might take weeks and even months. The intraocular pressure should be closed monitored during the episode. It should be noted that epithelialization does not necessary means that the ulcer is healing. In fact it might hinder the penetration of the fungicide. Confocal microscopy might be an effective additional method to follow the success or failure of the therapy. It does so by direct examination of the organism, inflammation, and corneal stromal cells.

Surgery

Periodic debridement is commonly used in the management fungal keratitis. The procedure removes necrotic tissue and diminishes the organism load but mostly it enhances the penetration of the drugs. It can be performed every 24 to 48 hours.

If everything fails, a conjunctival flap might deter the infection. If there is no response, then a lamellar or penetrating keratoplasty could be needed. If there is a perforation, a patch graft or a therapeutic transplant should be performed. The infected cornea should be sent for cultures and pathological evaluation. It is performed in the usual manner but it should extend about 1 to 1.5mm beyond the margins of the lesion.

Surgical Follow Up

Close follow up for at least 2 weeks with topical antimycotics is recommended. Systemic medication may be added as well. If the edges of the specimen are found by pathology to have organisms the use of topical and systemic antifungals should be extended.

Complications

Adverse results range from mild to severe corneal scarring, corneal perforation, anterior segment disruption and glaucoma to endophthalmitis resulting in evisceration.

Prognosis

The aftermath of fungal keratitis can be dismal . There is severe visual loss in 26% to 63% of patients. Fifteen to twenty percent may need evisceration. Penetrating keratoplasty is required in 31 to 38% of cases.

Otomycosis

Otomycosis is a fungal infection in the outer ear. An otomycosis infection causes inflammation, dry skin, and a smelly discharge in the ear canal.

People most likely to be affected by otomycosis include those who live in warm, tropical climates, and those who participate in water sports. Otomycosis is often easily treated with topical antifungal medications.

In this article, we look closely at otomycosis, including its causes, symptoms, treatment, and prevention.

Causes

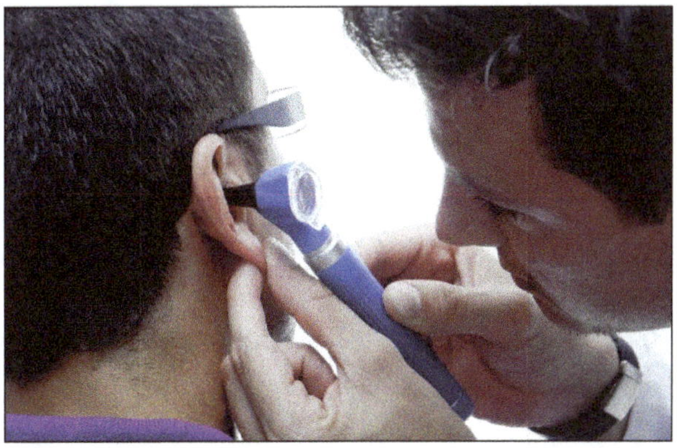

Otomycosis can cause hearing loss and a feeling of fullness in the ear.

Otomycosis is an infection caused by a fungus. There are several different types of fungus that can cause this infection, but most otomycosis infections are related to *Aspergillus* species or, less commonly, *Candida*.

People come into contact with fungi every day in the environment, but fungi do not typically pose a problem.

However, those with weakened immune systems can catch an infection more easily than others when they come into contact with a fungus.

Also, people who live in hot or tropical climates are more likely to experience otomycosis, as fungi thrive in warm, damp places.

Other risk factors include:

- Trauma to the ear from hearing aids or cotton swabs.
- Chronic skin conditions, such as eczema.
- Having diabetes mellitus.
- Participating in water sports, including swimming or surfing.
- Swimming in contaminated water.
- Lack of cerumen, or earwax, which suppresses bacterial or fungal growth and stops the ear canal drying out.

Symptoms

Typical symptoms of otomycosis include:

- Hearing loss, which can be mistaken for deafness.
- A feeling of fullness in the ear.
- Redness of the outer ear.
- Itching, a more common symptom of fungal infections than bacterial ones.
- Pain.
- Inflammation or swelling.
- Flaky skin.
- Ringing in the ears.
- Discharge from the ear, which can be white, yellow, gray, black, or green.

These symptoms typically occur in one ear, but it is possible that both ears can be affected at the same time.

Diagnosis

Symptoms of otomycosis should always be evaluated by a doctor in order to get the correct diagnosis and treatment.

The doctor will take a thorough medical history to determine if any risk factors are present. They will perform a physical exam with an instrument called an otoscope to look inside the ear canal and eardrum.

The doctor may also take a sample of cells or fluid from the ear and look at them under a microscope. This will help them to differentiate between a fungal or bacterial infection.

Treatment

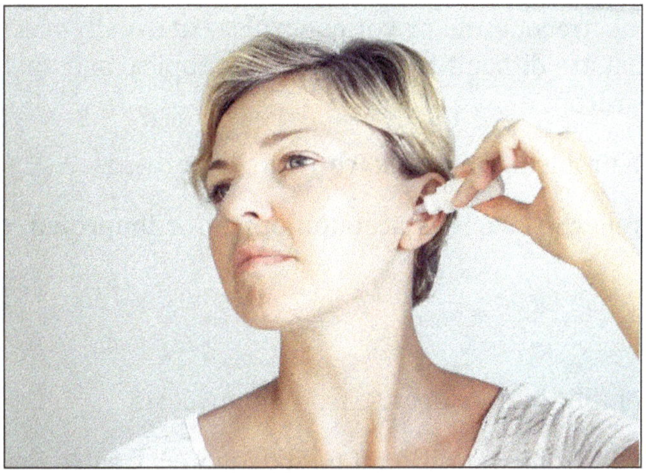

Eardrops may help to cure the infection and prevent it from reoccurring.

A doctor will prescribe the correct treatment once a diagnosis of otomycosis is made. Treatment can be eardrops, topical cream, or oral medication.

Cleaning

Firstly, a doctor usually needs to clean the ear. They may use a rinse or a suction tool to do this. Cleaning will get rid of debris or a buildup of material and allow the medication to work better.

Next, the ear is cleaned and dried, as much as possible, to inhibit further growth of fungus.

Note that a person should not attempt to clean their own ears with cotton swabs or other tools, as this could worsen the situation.

Eardrops or Topical Agents

A doctor may prescribe eardrops that contain an antifungal agent.

Research has shown that 1 percent clotrimazole eardrops show high rates of cure and prevention of recurrence.

Eardrops may also contain econazole, miconazole, or amphotericin B, among other chemicals.

Antifungals may also be in the form of a topical cream that is applied to the outer ear.

Other topical medications might include:

- Aluminum acetate.
- Salicylic acid.
- Hydrogen peroxide.

These agents can help to treat the fungus or soften the crust that forms to help other medications penetrate better.

Oral Medications

Oral medications, such as itraconazole or voriconazole, are usually reserved for more severe infections, or infections that are difficult to get rid of with topical agents. Some fungus species are resistant to antifungal eardrops.

Oral antifungals can be a problem for people who have liver disease.

Over-the-counter pain relievers, such as acetaminophen or ibuprofen, can be used to ease any minor pain.

Complications

Although uncommon, complications can arise from otomycosis.

Otomycosis can become a chronic condition if not adequately treated, or if it does not respond to treatment. This can also happen if a person has continued exposure to contaminated water that contains a fungus.

Otomycosis can invade further than the outer ear and perforate the eardrum or travel to places that may include the inner ear or base of the skull.

These types of infections typically require oral antifungal treatment and surgical management. A complication such as this is more likely to occur in those who have a weakened immune system or diabetes mellitus.

Prevention

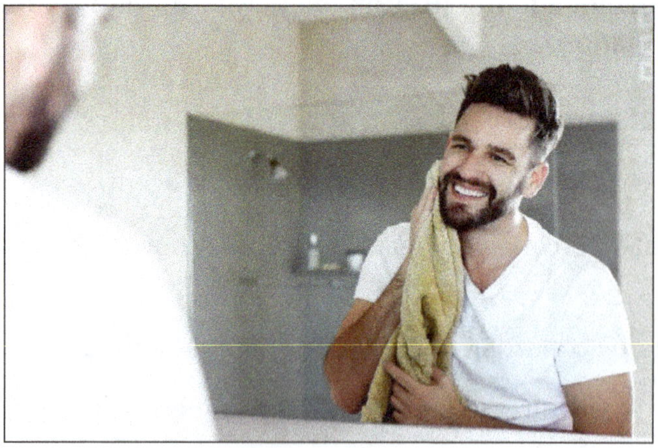

Drying the ears thoroughly after swimming and bathing can help to prevent otmycosis.

There are a few factors that can help prevent otomycosis, including:

- Leaving a small amount of earwax in the ears for its natural anti-fungal properties.
- Drying the ears well after swimming and bathing.
- Using earplugs when swimming to keep water out.

- Using a hairdryer on low speed to dry ears, being careful not to burn the skin.
- Avoiding scratching the ears as this may damage the skin and make it easier for a fungus to invade.
- Avoiding putting cotton swabs in the ears.

Aspergillosis

Aspergillosis is an infection caused by a type of mold (fungus). The illnesses resulting from aspergillosis infection usually affect the respiratory system, but their signs and severity vary greatly.

The mold that triggers the illnesses, aspergillus, is everywhere — indoors and outdoors. Most strains of this mold are harmless, but a few can cause serious illnesses when people with weakened immune systems, underlying lung disease or asthma inhale their fungal spores.

In some people, the spores trigger an allergic reaction. Other people develop mild to serious lung infections. The most serious form of aspergillosis — invasive aspergillosis — occurs when the infection spreads to blood vessels and beyond.

Depending on the type of aspergillosis, treatment may involve observation, antifungal medications or, in rare cases, surgery.

Symptoms

The signs and symptoms of aspergillosis vary with the type of illness you develop:

Allergic Reaction

Some people with asthma or cystic fibrosis have an allergic reaction to aspergillus mold. Signs and symptoms of this condition, known as allergic bronchopulmonary aspergillosis, include:

- Fever.
- A cough that may bring up blood or plugs of mucus.
- Worsening asthma.

Aspergilloma

Certain chronic lung (pulmonary) conditions, such as emphysema, tuberculosis or advanced sarcoidosis, can cause air spaces (cavities) to form in the lungs. When people with lung cavities are also infected with aspergillus, fungus fibers may find their way into the cavities and grow into tangled masses (fungus balls) known as aspergillomas.

Aspergillomas may produce no symptoms or cause only a mild cough at first. Over time and without treatment, however, aspergillomas can worsen the underlying chronic lung condition and possibly cause:

- A cough that often brings up blood (hemoptysis).
- Wheezing.
- Shortness of breath.
- Unintentional weight loss.
- Fatigue.

Invasive Aspergillosis

This is the most severe form of aspergillosis. It occurs when the infection spreads rapidly from the lungs to the brain, heart, kidneys or skin. Invasive aspergillosis occurs only in people whose immune systems are weakened as a result of cancer chemotherapy, bone marrow transplantation or a disease of the immune system. Untreated, this form of aspergillosis may be fatal.

Signs and symptoms depend on which organs are affected, but in general, invasive aspergillosis can cause:

- Fever and chills.
- A cough that brings up blood (hemoptysis).
- Shortness of breath.
- Chest or joint pain.
- Headaches or eye symptoms.
- Skin lesions.

Other Types of Aspergillosis

Aspergillus can invade areas of your body other than your lungs, such as your sinuses. In your sinuses, the fungus can cause a stuffy nose sometimes accompanied by drainage that may contain blood. Fever, facial pain and headache may also occur.

Doctor Consultation

If you have asthma or cystic fibrosis, see your doctor whenever you notice a change in your breathing. Although aspergillosis may not be the cause, it's important to have breathing problems evaluated.

If you have a weakened immune system and develop an unexplained fever, shortness of breath or a cough that brings up blood, get immediate medical care. In the case of invasive aspergillosis, prompt treatment is crucial. In some cases, treatment with antifungal medication begins as soon as aspergillosis is suspected, even before testing has confirmed the diagnosis.

Causes

Aspergillus mold is unavoidable. Outdoors, it's found in decaying leaves and compost and on plants, trees and grain crops.

Everyday exposure to aspergillus is rarely a problem for people with healthy immune systems. When mold spores are inhaled, immune system cells surround and destroy them. But people who have a weakened immune system from illness or immunosuppressant medications have fewer infection-fighting cells. This allows aspergillus to take hold, invading the lungs and, in the most serious cases, other parts of the body.

Aspergillosis is not contagious from person to person.

Risk Factors

Your risk of developing aspergillosis depends on your overall health and the extent of your exposure to mold. In general, these factors make you more vulnerable to infection:

- Weakened immune system: People taking immune-suppressing drugs after undergoing transplant surgery — especially bone marrow or stem cell transplants — or people who have certain cancers of the blood are at highest risk of invasive aspergillosis. People in the later stages of AIDS also may be at increased risk.
- Low white blood cell level: People who have had chemotherapy, an organ transplant or leukemia have lower white cell levels, making them more susceptible to invasive aspergillosis. So does having chronic granulomatous disease — an inherited disorder that affects immune system cells.
- Lung cavities: People who have air spaces (cavities) in their lungs are at higher risk of developing aspergillomas.
- Asthma or cystic fibrosis: People with asthma and cystic fibrosis, especially those whose lung problems are long-standing or hard to control, are more likely to have an allergic response to aspergillus mold.
- Long-term corticosteroid therapy: Long-term use of corticosteroids may increase the risk of opportunistic infections, depending on the underlying disease being treated and what other drugs are being used.

Complications

Depending on the type of infection, aspergillosis can cause a variety of serious complications:

- Bleeding: Both aspergillomas and invasive aspergillosis can cause severe, and sometimes fatal, bleeding in your lungs.
- Systemic infection: The most serious complication of invasive aspergillosis is the spread of the infection to other parts of your body, especially your brain, heart and kidneys. Invasive aspergillosis spreads rapidly and may be fatal.

Prevention

It's nearly impossible to avoid exposure to aspergillus, but if you have had a transplant or are undergoing chemotherapy, try to stay away from places where you're likely to encounter mold, such as construction sites, compost piles and buildings that store grain. If you have a weakened immune system, your doctor may advise you to wear a face mask to avoid being exposed to aspergillus and other airborne infectious agents.

Chapter 5

Antifungal Drugs: Types and Uses

Antifungal Drugs

Antifungal medicines or drugs are used to treat fungal infections.

Amphoterecin B

Amphotericin B is used in the treatment of severe fungal infections and kala-azar.

Working of Amphotericin B

Amphotericin B is an antifungal medication. It kills fungi by destroying the fungal cell membrane.

Common Side Effects of Amphotericin B

Nausea, Vomiting, Chills, Headache, Anemia (low number of red blood cells), Decreased potassium level in blood, Abnormal liver function tests, Decreased magnesium level in blood, Diarrhea, Decreased appetite, Hypotension (low blood pressure), Skin rash, Nephrocalcinosis, Increased creatinine level in blood, Abnormal renal function tests, and Renal tubular acidosis.

- It is usually given as an injection over 1-2 hours under the supervision of a medical professional.
- Amphotericin B can cause rash, chills, headache, and tiredness during initial days of the treatment, but these may fade away with time.
- Your doctor may ask you for regular blood tests to monitor your blood sugar, potassium, magnesium and kidney function.
- Inform your doctor immediately if you notice pain or blood upon urination, swelling of the face and trouble breathing.
- Inform your doctor if you are pregnant, planning pregnancy or breastfeeding.

Amphotericin B is an antifungal antibiotic for the treatment of serious infections caused by fungi like fungal infections of one or more deep organs of the body, suspected fungal infections in patients with a raised temperature and neutropenia (reduced number of white blood cells [neutrophils]) and Visceral leishmaniasis (disease caused by a parasite). It is light insensitive.

Liposomal Amphotericin B is a lipid-associated formulation. Liposomal encapsulation or incorporation into a lipid complex of Amphotericin B can substantially improves drug safety especially nephrotoxicity associated with the drug.

Administration of Amphotericin B is associated with allergy (severe and serious allergic) reaction, therefore it is recommended to administer a test dose before starting the therapy to check for sensitivity. Amphotericin B is either administered as intravenous injection or infusion by a registered medical professional only. Amphotericin B can disrupt the lipid components of human kidney cells, thereby causing nephrotoxicity. The exact mechanism of hypokalemia is not known, but kidney damage may result in excessive loss of potassium in urine.

Fluconazole

Fluconazole is used to prevent and treat a variety of fungal and yeast infections. It belongs to a class of drugs called azole antifungals. It works by stopping the growth of certain types of fungus.

Guidelines to use Fluconazole

Read the Patient Information Leaflet if available from your pharmacist before you start taking fluconazole and each time you get a refill. If you have any questions, ask your doctor or pharmacist.

Take this medication by mouth with or without food as directed by your doctor, usually once daily.

If you are taking the liquid suspension form of this medication, shake the bottle well before each dose. Carefully measure the dose using a special measuring device/spoon. Do not use a household spoon because you may not get the correct dose.

Dosage is based on your medical condition and response to treatment. For children, dosage is also based on weight. Generally in children, the dose should not exceed 600 milligrams daily unless directed by the doctor. This medication works best when the amount of medicine in your body is kept at a constant level. Take it at the same time each day as directed.

Continue to take this medication until the full prescribed amount is finished, even if symptoms disappear after a few days. Stopping the medication too early may allow the fungus to continue to grow, which may result in a return of the infection. Tell your doctor if your condition lasts or gets worse.

Nausea, vomiting, diarrhea, stomach upset/pain, headache, dizziness, or hair loss may occur. If any of these effects last or get worse, tell your doctor or pharmacist promptly.

Remember that this medication has been prescribed because your doctor has judged that the benefit to you is greater than the risk of side effects. Many people using this medication do not have serious side effects.

Tell your doctor right away if you have any serious side effects, including: signs of your adrenal glands not working well (such as loss of appetite, unusual tiredness, weight loss).

Get medical help right away if you have any very serious side effects, including: fast/irregular heartbeat, severe dizziness, fainting.

This drug may rarely cause serious liver disease. Get medical help right away if you develop any signs of liver disease, including: nausea/vomiting that doesn't stop, severe stomach/abdominal pain, yellowing eyes/skin, dark urine.

A very serious allergic reaction to this drug is rare. However, get medical help right away if you notice any symptoms of a serious allergic reaction, including: fever that doesn't go away, new or worsening lymph node swelling, rash, itching/swelling (especially of the face/tongue/throat), severe dizziness, trouble breathing.

This is not a complete list of possible side effects. If you notice other effects not listed above, contact your doctor or pharmacist.

Itraconazole

Itraconazole is used to treat serious fungal or yeast infections. Itraconazole oral solution is only used to treat oropharyngeal or esophageal candidiasis (thrush, oral thrush). Itraconazole capsule is used to treat fungal infections, such as aspergillosis (fungal infection in the lungs), blastomycosis (Gilchrist's disease), or histoplasmosis (Darling's disease). Sporanox® capsule is also used to treat onychomycosis (fungal infection in the fingernails or toenails). Itraconazole tablet is only used to treat onychomycosis of the toenails. This medicine works by killing the fungus or yeast and preventing its growth.

This medicine is available only with your doctor's prescription.

This product is available in the following dosage forms:

- Capsule
- Solution

Precautions before using Itraconazole

In deciding to use a medicine, the risks of taking the medicine must be weighed against the good it will do. This is a decision you and your doctor will make. For this medicine, the following should be considered:

Allergies

Tell your doctor if you have ever had any unusual or allergic reaction to this medicine or any other medicines. Also tell your health care professional if you have any other types of allergies, such as to foods, dyes, preservatives, or animals. For non-prescription products, read the label or package ingredients carefully.

Pediatric

Appropriate studies on the relationship of age to the effects of itraconazole have not been performed in the pediatric population. Safety and efficacy have not been established.

Geriatric

Appropriate studies performed to date have not demonstrated geriatric-specific problems that would limit the usefulness of itraconazole in the elderly. However, elderly patients are more likely to have temporary or permanent hearing loss or age-related kidney, liver, or heart problems, which may require caution and an adjustment in the dose for patients receiving itraconazole.

Breastfeeding

There are no adequate studies in women for determining infant risk when using this medication during breastfeeding. Weigh the potential benefits against the potential risks before taking this medication while breastfeeding.

Drug Interactions

Although certain medicines should not be used together at all, in other cases two different medicines may be used together even if an interaction might occur. In these cases, your doctor may want to change the dose, or other precautions may be necessary. When you are taking this medicine, it is especially important that your healthcare professional know if you are taking any of the medicines listed below. The following interactions have been selected on the basis of their potential significance and are not necessarily all-inclusive.

Using this medicine with any of the following medicines is not recommended. Your doctor may decide not to treat you with this medication or change some of the other medicines you take.

- Alfuzosin
- Alprazolam
- Astemizole
- Avanafil
- Bepridil
- Cisapride
- Colchicine
- Conivaptan
- Dabigatran Etexilate
- Dihydroergotamine
- Disopyramide
- Dofetilide
- Dronedarone
- Eletriptan
- Eliglustat
- Eplerenone

- Ergonovine
- Ergotamine
- Felodipine
- Finerenone
- Flibanserin
- Fluconazole
- Irinotecan
- Irinotecan Liposome
- Isavuconazonium Sulfate
- Ivabradine
- Levoketoconazole
- Levomethadyl
- Lomitapide
- Lovastatin
- Lurasidone
- Maraviroc
- Mavacamten
- Mesoridazine
- Methadone
- Methylergonovine
- Methysergide
- Midazolam
- Naloxegol
- Nelfinavir
- Nisoldipine
- Pacritinib
- Pimozide
- Piperaquine

- Posaconazole
- Quinidine
- Ranolazine
- Silodosin
- Simvastatin
- Solifenacin
- Sparfloxacin
- Telithromycin
- Terfenadine
- Thioridazine
- Ticagrelor
- Tolvaptan
- Triazolam
- Ubrogepant
- Venetoclax
- Voclosporin
- Ziprasidone

Using this medicine with any of the following medicines is usually not recommended, but may be required in some cases. If both medicines are prescribed together, your doctor may change the dose or how often you use one or both of the medicines.

- Abametapir
- Acalabrutinib
- Adagrasib
- Ado-Trastuzumab Emtansine
- Afatinib
- Alfentanil
- Aliskiren
- Amiodarone
- Amisulpride

- Anagrelide
- Apalutamide
- Apixaban
- Apomorphine
- Aprepitant
- Aripiprazole
- Aripiprazole Lauroxil
- Arsenic Trioxide
- Asciminib
- Atogepant
- Atorvastatin
- Avacopan
- Avapritinib
- Axitinib
- Bedaquiline
- Benzhydrocodone
- Berotralstat
- Betrixaban
- Boceprevir
- Bosutinib
- Bretylium
- Brexpiprazole
- Brigatinib
- Bromocriptine
- Budesonide
- Buprenorphine
- Buserelin
- Cabazitaxel

- Cabozantinib
- Calcifediol
- Carbamazepine
- Cariprazine
- Ceritinib
- Chloroquine
- Cilostazol
- Citalopram
- Clarithromycin
- Clofazimine
- Clothiapine
- Clozapine
- Cobicistat
- Cobimetinib
- Codeine
- Copanlisib
- Crizotinib
- Cyclosporine
- Dabrafenib
- Daclatasvir
- Daridorexant
- Darifenacin
- Dasatinib
- Deflazacort
- Degarelix
- Delamanid
- Deslorelin
- Deutetrabenazine

- Dexamethasone
- Dexmedetomidine
- Digoxin
- Dihydrocodeine
- Docetaxel
- Domperidone
- Donepezil
- Doxorubicin
- Doxorubicin Hydrochloride Liposome
- Duvelisib
- Edoxaban
- Efavirenz
- Elagolix
- Elbasvir
- Elexacaftor
- Elvitegravir
- Encorafenib
- Entrectinib
- Erlotinib
- Escitalopram
- Eszopiclone
- Everolimus
- Fedratinib
- Fentanyl
- Fesoterodine
- Fexinidazole
- Fingolimod
- Fluoxetine

- Fluticasone
- Formoterol
- Fosaprepitant
- Foscarnet
- Fosnetupitant
- Fosphenytoin
- Fostemsavir
- Futibatinib
- Gilteritinib
- Glasdegib
- Gonadorelin
- Goserelin
- Grazoprevir
- Halofantrine
- Haloperidol
- Histrelin
- Hydrocodone
- Hydroxychloroquine
- Hydroxyzine
- Ibrexafungerp
- Ibrutinib
- Ibutilide
- Idelalisib
- Iloperidone
- Infigratinib
- Inotuzumab Ozogamicin
- Istradefylline
- Ivacaftor

- Ivosidenib
- Ixabepilone
- Lapatinib
- Larotrectinib
- Lefamulin
- Lemborexant
- Lenvatinib
- Leuprolide
- Levofloxacin
- Levomilnacipran
- Lofexidine
- Lorlatinib
- Lumacaftor
- Lumateperone
- Lurbinectedin
- Macimorelin
- Macitentan
- Manidipine
- Meperidine
- Metronidazole
- Midostaurin
- Mifepristone
- Mirtazapine
- Mirvetuximab Soravtansine-gynx
- Mitapivat
- Mobocertinib
- Morphine
- Morphine Sulfate Liposome

- Moxifloxacin
- Nafarelin
- Neratinib
- Netupitant
- Nevirapine
- Nifedipine
- Nilotinib
- Olaparib
- Ondansetron
- Osilodrostat
- Osimertinib
- Oxaliplatin
- Oxycodone
- Ozanimod
- Palbociclib
- Panobinostat
- Pasireotide
- Pazopanib
- Pemigatinib
- Pentazocine
- Pexidartinib
- Phenytoin
- Pimavanserin
- Pitolisant
- Pixantrone
- Ponatinib
- Ponesimod
- Pralsetinib

- Quetiapine
- Reboxetine
- Regorafenib
- Relugolix
- Repaglinide
- Retapamulin
- Ribociclib
- Rifabutin
- Rifampin
- Rimegepant
- Riociguat
- Risperidone
- Rivaroxaban
- Romidepsin
- Ruxolitinib
- Salmeterol
- Selpercatinib
- Selumetinib
- Sertraline
- Sevoflurane
- Sildenafil
- Simeprevir
- Siponimod
- Sirolimus
- Sirolimus Protein-Bound
- Sonidegib
- Sotalol
- St John's Wort

- Sufentanil
- Sulpiride
- Sunitinib
- Suvorexant
- Tacrolimus
- Tadalafil
- Talazoparib
- Tamsulosin
- Tazemetostat
- Temsirolimus
- Tezacaftor
- Thiotepa
- Topotecan
- Toremifene
- Trabectedin
- Tramadol
- Trazodone
- Triclabendazole
- Triptorelin
- Upadacitinib
- Valbenazine
- Vandetanib
- Vardenafil
- Vemurafenib
- Venlafaxine
- Vilanterol
- Vilazodone
- Vinblastine

- Vincristine
- Vincristine Sulfate Liposome
- Vinflunine
- Vinorelbine
- Vorapaxar
- Warfarin
- Zanubrutinib
- Zolpidem
- Zuclopenthixol

Using this medicine with any of the following medicines may cause an increased risk of certain side effects, but using both drugs may be the best treatment for you. If both medicines are prescribed together, your doctor may change the dose or how often you use one or both of the medicines.

- Acenocoumarol
- Amlodipine
- Anisindione
- Buspirone
- Busulfan
- Ciprofloxacin
- Dicumarol
- Didanosine
- Indinavir
- Meloxicam
- Micafungin
- Nirmatrelvir
- Phenprocoumon
- Ritonavir
- Rosuvastatin
- Saquinavir
- Tolterodine

Other Interactions

Certain medicines should not be used at or around the time of eating food or eating certain types of food since interactions may occur. Using alcohol or tobacco with certain medicines may also cause interactions to occur. The following interactions have been selected on the basis of their potential significance and are not necessarily all-inclusive.

Using this medicine with any of the following may cause an increased risk of certain side effects but may be unavoidable in some cases. If used together, your doctor may change the dose or how often you use this medicine, or give you special instructions about the use of food, alcohol, or tobacco.

- Food
- Grapefruit Juice

Other Medical Problems

The presence of other medical problems may affect the use of this medicine. Make sure you tell your doctor if you have any other medical problems, especially:

- Chronic obstructive pulmonary disease (COPD) or
- Edema (body swelling or fluid retention) or
- Heart attack, history of or
- Heart disease (e.g., ischemic disease, valve problems) or
- Heart rhythm problems—Use with caution. May increase the risk for more serious side effects.
- Congestive heart failure—Use with caution. Tolsura™ may make this condition worse.
- Congestive heart failure or history of—Should not be used to treat fungal infection of the fingernails or toenails in patients with this condition.
- Cystic fibrosis or
- Hypochlorhydria (low level of acid in the stomach) in HIV-infected patients or
- Patients who have had an organ transplant—Absorption from the stomach may change.
- Elevated liver enzymes or
- Kidney disease or
- Liver disease, active or history of—Use with caution. May make these conditions worse.

Proper use

Take this medicine only as directed by your doctor. Do not take more of it, do not take it more often, and do not take it for a longer time than your doctor ordered.

This medicine comes with a patient information leaflet. Read and follow the instructions carefully. Ask your doctor if you have any questions.

Keep using this medicine for the full treatment time, even if you feel better after the first few doses. Your infection may not clear up if you stop using the medicine too soon.

Itraconazole capsules and tablets should be taken with a full meal. The oral liquid is best taken on an empty stomach. Take the tablets at the same time each day.

Measure the oral liquid with a marked measuring spoon or medicine cup. If you have thrush in the mouth or throat, place 10 milliliters (mL) of the liquid in your mouth, swish for several seconds, then swallow. Repeat these steps if your total dose is more than 10 mL.

If you are using antacids (e.g., Maalox®, Mylanta®, Pepcid® Complete, Rolaids®, or Tums®) or other stomach medicine (e.g., H2 blocker, proton pump inhibitor), take them at least 2 hours before or 2 hours after using itraconazole. You may also take itraconazole with an acidic beverage (e.g., non-diet cola) if you are taking it with an antacid.

Use only the brand and the dosage form of this medicine that your doctor prescribed. Different brands and dosage forms may not work the same way.

Sporanox® oral liquid works differently than itraconazole Sporanox® capsules, even at the same dose (number of milligrams). Do not switch from the capsules to the oral liquid unless your doctor tells you to.

Dosing

The dose of this medicine will be different for different patients. Follow your doctor's orders or the directions on the label. The following information includes only the average doses of this medicine. If your dose is different, do not change it unless your doctor tells you to do so.

The amount of medicine that you take depends on the strength of the medicine. Also, the number of doses you take each day, the time allowed between doses, and the length of time you take the medicine depend on the medical problem for which you are using the medicine.

- For oral dosage form (capsules):
    - For aspergillosis:
        - Adults:
            - Sporanox®—200 to 400 milligrams (mg) per day.
            - Tolsura™—130 mg (two capsules) once or 2 times a day.
            - Children—Use and dose must be determined by your doctor.
    - For blastomycosis or histoplasmosis:
        - Adults:
            - Sporanox®—200 milligrams (mg) (two capsules) once a day. Your doctor may

increase your dose as needed. However, the dose is usually not more than 400 mg per day.

        - Tolsura™—130 mg (two capsules) once a day. Your doctor may increase your dose as needed. However, the dose is usually not more than 260 mg per day.
      - Children—Use and dose must be determined by your doctor.
    - For onychomycosis of the fingernails:
      - Adults—200 milligrams (mg) 2 times a day for 1 week, followed by a no treatment period of 3 weeks, then 200 mg 2 times a day for 1 week.
      - Children—Use and dose must be determined by your doctor.
    - For onychomycosis of the toenails:
      - Adults—200 milligrams (mg) once a day for 12 weeks in a row.
      - Children—Use and dose must be determined by your doctor.
- For oral dosage form (liquid):
    - For esophageal candidiasis:
      - Adults—100 milligrams (mg) or 10 milliliters (mL) once a day for a minimum of 3 weeks. Your doctor may increase your dose as needed.
      - Children—Use and dose must be determined by your doctor.
    - For oropharyngeal candidiasis:
      - Adults—200 milligrams (mg) or 20 milliliters (mL) once a day for 1 to 2 weeks.
      - Children—Use and dose must be determined by your doctor.
- For oral dosage form (tablets):
    - For onychomycosis of the toenails:
      - Adults—200 milligrams (mg) once a day for 12 weeks in a row.
      - Children—Use and dose must be determined by your doctor.

Missed Dose

If you have missed your scheduled dose call your doctor or pharmacist for instructions.

Storage

Store the medicine in a closed container at room temperature, away from heat, moisture, and direct light. Keep from freezing.

Keep out of the reach of children.

Do not keep outdated medicine or medicine no longer needed. Ask your healthcare professional how you should dispose of any medicine you do not use.

Precautions

It is very important that your doctor check your progress at regular visits to make sure that this medicine is working properly. Blood tests may be needed to check for unwanted effects.

If your symptoms do not improve, or if they become worse, check with your doctor. You may need to take this medicine for several weeks or months before your infection gets better.

Do not use avanafil (Stendra™), cisapride (Propulsid®), disopyramide (Norpace®), dofetilide (Tikosyn®), dronedarone (Multaq®), eliglustat (Cerdelga™), eplerenone (Inspra®), felodipine (Plendil®), irinotecan (Camptosar®), isavuconazole (Cresemba®), ivabradine (Corlanor®), lomitapide (Juxtapid™), lurasidone (Latuda®), methadone (Dolophine®), naloxegol (Movantik®), nisoldipine (Sular®), oral midazolam (Versed®), pimozide (Orap®), quinidine (Cardioquin®, Quinaglute®), ranolazine (Ranexa®), ticagrelor (Brilinta®), triazolam (Halcion®), venetoclax (Venclexta®), an ergot medicine (e.g., dihydroergotamine, ergometrine, ergotamine, methylergometrine, Cafergot®, Ergomar®, Wigraine®), or certain medicines to lower cholesterol (e.g., lovastatin, simvastatin, Mevacor®, Zocor®) during and 2 weeks after treatment with itraconazole. Do not use colchicine (Colcrys®), fesoterodine (Toviaz®), solifenacin (Vesicare®), or telithromycin (Ketek®) during and 2 weeks after treatment with itraconazole, if you have kidney or liver disease. Using these medicines together may increase your risk for serious side effects.

Make sure your doctor knows if you are pregnant or planning to get pregnant before you start using this medicine for a fingernail or toenail infection. The capsule or tablet should not be used to treat onychomycosis in pregnant women or those who are planning to get pregnant. Use a highly effective form of birth control while you are using this medicine and for 2 months after your last dose. If you think you have become pregnant while using the medicine, tell your doctor right away.

Check with your doctor right away if you are having chest pain or tightness, decreased urine output, dilated neck veins, extreme fatigue, irregular breathing, an irregular heartbeat, swelling of the face, fingers, feet, or lower legs, trouble breathing, or weight gain. These could be symptoms of a side effect called congestive heart failure.

Rarely, this medicine may cause severe liver problems. Check with your doctor right away if you have stomach pain or tenderness, clay-colored stools, dark urine, decreased appetite, fever, headache, itching, loss of appetite, nausea, vomiting, skin rash, swelling of the feet or lower legs, unusual tiredness or weakness, or yellow eyes or skin.

This medicine may cause nerve problems. Call your doctor right away if your skin feels like it is burning, crawling, itching, or if you have numbness, prickling, "pins and needles", or a tingling feeling after using itraconazole.

Temporary or permanent hearing loss may occur while you are using this medicine. Check with your doctor right away if you have any changes in your hearing.

This medicine may make you feel dizzy or have blurred or double vision. Do not drive or do anything else that could be dangerous until you know how this medicine affects you.

Do not take other medicines unless they have been discussed with your doctor. This includes prescription or nonprescription (over-the-counter [OTC]) medicines and herbal or vitamin supplements.

Side Effects

Along with its needed effects, a medicine may cause some unwanted effects. Although not all of these side effects may occur, if they do occur they may need medical attention. Check with your doctor immediately if any of the following side effects occur:

More Common

- Decreased urine output,
- Dry mouth,
- Fever,
- Increased thirst,
- Irregular heartbeat,
- Loss of appetite,
- Mood changes,
- Muscle pain or cramps,
- Nausea,
- Numbness or tingling in the hands, feet, or lips,
- Seizures,
- Trouble breathing,
- Unusual tiredness or weakness, and
- Vomiting.

Less Common

- Blurred vision,
- Chest pain,
- Chills,
- Clay-colored stools,
- Cloudy urine,
- Cold sweats,

- Confusion,
- Cough,
- Dark urine,
- Decrease in urine-concentrating ability,
- Diarrhea,
- Dizziness,
- Dizziness, faintness, or lightheadedness when getting up suddenly from a lying or sitting position,
- Drowsiness,
- Feeling unusually cold,
- Headache,
- Itching, skin rash,
- Light-colored stools,
- Mental changes,
- Muscle cramps in the hands, arms, feet, legs, or face,
- Muscle spasms (tetany) or twitching,
- Nervousness,
- Noisy, rattling breathing,
- Numbness and tingling around the mouth or fingertips,
- Pounding in the ears,
- Shivering,
- Slow, fast, or pounding heartbeat or pulse,
- Sneezing,
- Sore throat,
- Stomach cramps or pain,
- Sweating,
- Swelling of the fingers, hands, feet, or lower legs,
- Tightness in the chest,

- Trembling,
- Trouble breathing at rest,
- Unpleasant breath odor,
- Vomiting of blood,
- Weight gain, and
- Yellow eyes or skin.

Rare

- Black, tarry stools,
- Bleeding gums,
- Blistering, peeling, or loosening of the skin,
- Bloating or swelling of the face, arms, hands, lower legs, or feet,
- Blood in the urine or stools,
- Blue lips and fingernails,
- Burning, crawling, itching, numbness, painful, prickling, “pins and needles”, or tingling feelings,
- Continuing ringing or buzzing or other unexplained noise in the ears,
- Coughing that sometimes produces a pink frothy sputum,
- Cracks in the skin,
- Decreased appetite,
- Difficulty with swallowing,
- Dilated neck veins,
- Disturbed color perception,
- Double vision,
- Extreme tiredness or weakness,
- Fast or irregular breathing,
- Feeling of discomfort,
- General feeling of tiredness or weakness,
- Halos around lights,

- Hearing loss,
- Hives or welts,
- Inflammation of the joints,
- Joint pain,
- Large, hive-like swelling on the face, eyelids, lips, tongue, throat, hands, legs, feet, or genitals,
- Loss of heat from the body,
- Loss of vision,
- Lower back or side pain,
- Night blindness,
- Overbright appearance of lights,
- Painful or difficult urination,
- Pale skin,
- Pinpoint red spots on the skin,
- Puffiness or swelling of the eyelids or around the eyes, face, lips, or tongue,
- Rapid weight gain,
- Red skin lesions, often with a purple center,
- Red, irritated eyes,
- Red, swollen skin,
- Scaly skin,
- Sores, ulcers, or white spots on the lips or in the mouth,
- Stomach pain, continuing,
- Stomach tenderness,
- Swollen lymph glands,
- Tunnel vision,
- Unsteadiness or awkwardness,
- Unusual bleeding or bruising,
- Unusual weight gain or loss,

- Upper right abdominal or stomach pain, and
- Weakness in the arms, hands, legs, or feet.

Incidence not known

- Bloating,
- Constipation,
- Difficult, fast, noisy breathing,
- Indigestion,
- Loss of bladder control, and
- Pains in the stomach, side, or abdomen, possibly radiating to the back.

Some side effects may occur that usually do not need medical attention. These side effects may go away during treatment as your body adjusts to the medicine. Also, your health care professional may be able to tell you about ways to prevent or reduce some of these side effects. Check with your health care professional if any of the following side effects continue or are bothersome or if you have any questions about them:

Less Common

- Decreased interest in sexual intercourse,
- Difficulty having a bowel movement,
- Difficulty with moving,
- Discouragement,
- Feeling of constant movement of self or surroundings,
- Feeling sad or empty,
- Inability to have or keep an erection,
- Irritability,
- Loss in sexual ability, desire, drive, or performance,
- Loss of interest or pleasure,
- Muscle aching or stiffness,
- Pain or tenderness around the eyes and cheekbones,
- Passing of gas,
- Sensation of spinning,

- Sleepiness or unusual drowsiness,
- Soreness of the skin,
- Stomach fullness or discomfort,
- Stuffy or runny nose,
- Trouble concentrating, and
- Trouble sleeping.

Rare

- Belching,
- Change in taste,
- Hair loss or thinning of the hair,
- Heartburn,
- Increased need to urinate,
- Increased sensitivity of the eyes or skin to sunlight,
- Loss of taste,
- Menstrual changes,
- Passing urine more often,
- Redness or other discoloration of the skin, and
- Severe sunburn.

Ketoconazole

Ketoconazole is an antifungal medicine. It's used to treat skin infections caused by a fungus (yeast). It can also prevent them coming back.

It treats different types of fungal infections including:

- Athlete's foot,
- Jock itch, an infection in the groin area,
- Sweat rash (intertrigo), a rash that usually appears in folds of skin,
- Dandruff and seborrhoeic dermatitis, where your scalp or other areas of your skin become scaly and dry or greasy, and
- Pityriasis versicolor, sometimes called tinea versicolour, where small patches of skin become scaly and change colour.

Ketoconazole is available as a cream or shampoo. You can buy most ketoconazole creams and shampoos in pharmacies and supermarkets, or get them on prescription. For treating pityriasis versicolor, you will need a prescription.

Ketoconazole also comes as tablets but these usually only treat a rare condition called Cushing's syndrome. The tablets are available on prescription only, and they are not covered here.

Key Facts

- Ketoconazole usually works within 2 to 3 weeks for most fungal infections, but it can take 6 weeks for athlete's foot to get better.
- It works by killing the yeasts (fungi) that cause the infections.
- The most common side effects of the cream and shampoo are irritated or red skin.
- For most infections, you'll usually use the cream once or twice a day and the shampoo once or twice a week.
- Some people use ketoconazole shampoo every 1 to 2 weeks to help stop dandruff coming back.

Warnings

Ketoconazole creams and shampoos can be used by most adults and children aged 12 years and over.

Ketoconazole is not suitable for everyone. To make sure it's safe for you, talk to your doctor or pharmacist before using it if you have ever had an allergic reaction to ketoconazole or any other medicine.

Guidelines to use Ketoconazole

Always follow the instructions that come with your medicine, or your doctor's advice.

How long you use ketoconazole for and how often depend on the type of skin problem you have.

Using cream for Athlete'S Foot, Jock itch and Sweat Rash

Use the cream once or twice a day on the infected skin and surrounding area. For athlete's foot, you need to use it twice a day regularly.

Carry on using the cream for 3 days after your symptoms have cleared up, to stop the infection coming back.

Using Shampoo or Cream for Seborrhoeic Dermatitis

Use the shampoo twice a week for 2 to 4 weeks until your symptoms have cleared. Then use it once every 1 to 2 weeks, to stop them coming back.

Alternatively, you can use the cream once or twice a day, for 2 to 4 weeks, and then use the shampoo once every 1 to 2 weeks to stop your symptoms coming back.

Using Shampoo for Dandruff

Use the shampoo twice a week for 2 to 4 weeks, then once every 1 to 2 weeks to stop your dandruff coming back.

Using Cream or Shampoo for Pityriasis Versicolor

Use the shampoo once a day, for up to 5 days.

For treating small areas of skin, you can use the cream instead. Put the cream on once or twice a day for 2 to 3 weeks.

If your symptoms tend to return in sunlight, use the shampoo once a day for up to 3 days before going out in the sun.

Steps to use Ketoconazole Cream

1. Wash and dry the infected area of skin. If you're treating your feet, make sure you dry between your toes.
2. Use your own towel or flannel. This stops you passing the infection on to anyone else.
3. Gently rub the cream into the infected area and surrounding skin. You'll usually need a small amount, depending on the size of the area you're treating. Be careful not to let the cream get into your eyes or mouth. If it does get into your eyes or mouth, rinse them with water.
4. Wash your hands afterwards. This stops you spreading the infection to other parts of your body or other people.

If you're using any other creams, ointments or lotions on the same area of skin, do not put them on at the same time as ketoconazole cream. After putting on the ketoconazole cream, wait 30 minutes before you use different products on the same area. This gives the ketoconazole time to be absorbed into your skin.

Steps to use ketoconazole Shampoo

1. Rinse your hair or the infected area of skin with water.
2. Shake the shampoo bottle, then squeeze a small amount onto the infected area.
3. If you're treating your scalp, massage the shampoo into your scalp until it makes a lather.
4. Leave the shampoo on for 3 to 5 minutes, then wash it off with water. Try not to get the shampoo into your eyes or mouth. If it gets into your eyes or mouth, rinse them with water.
5. Wash your hands afterwards. This stops you spreading the infection to other parts of your body or other people.

Missed dose

If you forget to use your ketoconazole cream or shampoo, just skip the missed dose and then keep to your usual routine.

Excessive Use

If you use too much ketoconazole shampoo or cream, or use it more often than you need to, it may make your skin irritated or red. If this happens, use less the next time.

Side Effects of Ketoconazole

Like all medicines, ketoconazole cream and shampoo can cause side effects, but not everyone gets them. Most side effects are minor. You can try using a smaller amount of the cream or shampoo to see if that helps.

Common Side Effects

You're unlikely to have common side effects when using the right amount of ketoconazole shampoo.

With ketoconazole cream, common side effects happen in more than 1 in 100 people. They usually affect your skin where you've applied the cream.

Talk to a pharmacist or doctor if these side effects bother you or do not go away, or if they spread beyond the area of skin you've treated:

- Itching or redness, and
- A burning feeling on your skin.

Serious Allergic Reaction

Serious allergic reactions (anaphylaxis) are rare but can happen with ketoconazole cream or shampoo.

Handling Side Effects of Ketoconazole

If itching, redness, or a burning feeling on your skin persists – Try using less cream. Apply it carefully, just to the area you need to treat. Rub it in gently. Try wearing loose clothing to reduce sweat. If the itching, redness or burning feeling is no better after a few days, or it gets worse at any time, stop using the cream and speak to a pharmacist or doctor.

Pregnancy and Breastfeeding

Ketoconazole and Pregnancy

You can use ketoconazole cream or shampoo if you're pregnant. Only tiny amounts are absorbed into your body so it will not affect your baby.

Ketoconazole and Breastfeeding

If you want to breastfeed and are using ketoconazole on your chest, wash any cream off your breasts and nipples and then wash your hands before feeding your baby.

Voriconazole

Voriconazole is used in adults and children 2 years of age and older to treat serious fungal infections such as invasive aspergillosis (a fungal infection that begins in the lungs and spreads through the bloodstream to other organs), esophageal candidiasis (a yeast [a type of fungus] infection that may cause white patching in the mouth and throat), and candidemia (a fungal infection in the blood). It is also used to treat certain other fungal infections when other medications will not work for certain patients. Voriconazole is in a class of antifungal medications called triazoles. It works by slowing the growth of the fungi that cause infection.

Uses of Voriconazole

Voriconazole comes as a tablet and a suspension (liquid) to take by mouth. It is usually taken every 12 hours on an empty stomach, at least 1 hour before or 1 hour after a meal. To help you remember to take voriconazole, take it at around the same times every day. Follow the directions on your prescription label carefully, and ask your doctor or pharmacist to explain any part you do not understand. Take voriconazole exactly as directed. Do not take more or less of it or take it more often than prescribed by your doctor.

If you are taking voriconazole suspension, shake the closed bottle for about 10 seconds before each use to mix the medication evenly. Do not mix the suspension with any other medications, water, or any other liquid. Always use the measuring device that comes with your medication. You may not receive the correct amount of medication if you use a household spoon to measure your dose.

At the beginning of your treatment, you may receive voriconazole by intravenous (into a vein) injection. When you begin taking voriconazole by mouth, your doctor may start you on a low dose and increase your dose if your condition does not improve. Your doctor also may decrease your dose if you experience side effects from voriconazole.

The length of your treatment depends on your general health, the type of infection you have, and how well you respond to the medication. Continue to take voriconazole even if you feel well. Do not stop taking voriconazole without talking to your doctor.

Other uses for this Medicine

This medication may be prescribed for other uses; ask your doctor or pharmacist for more information.

Precautions

Before taking voriconazole,

- Tell your doctor and pharmacist if you are allergic to voriconazole, other antifungal medications such as fluconazole (Diflucan), itraconazole (Onmel, Sporanox), or ketoconazole (Nizoral);any other medications, lactose, or any of the other ingredients in voriconazole tablets and suspension. Ask your pharmacist for a list of the ingredients in voriconazole tablets and suspension.

- Some medications should not be taken with voriconazole. Make sure you have discussed any medications you are currently taking or plan to take before starting voriconazole with your doctor and pharmacist. Before starting, stopping or changing any medications while taking voriconazole, please get the advice of your doctor or pharmacist.
- The following nonprescription or herbal products may interact with voriconazole: fluticasone (Flonase), ibuprofen (Motrin), mometasone (Nasonex), omeprazole (Prilosec), St. John's Wort. Be sure to let your doctor and pharmacist know that you are taking these medications before you start taking voriconazole. Do not start these medications while taking voriconaole without discussing with your healthcare provider.
- Tell your doctor if you have ever been treated with chemotherapy medications for cancer, and if you have or have ever had a prolonged QT interval (a rare heart problem that may cause irregular heartbeat, fainting, or sudden death), or if you have or ever had a slow or irregular heartbeat, low blood levels of potassium, magnesium, or calcium, cardiomyopathy (enlarged or thickened heart muscle that stops the heart from pumping blood normally), cancer of the blood cells, galactose intolerance or glucose–galactose malabsorption (inherited conditions where the body is not able to tolerate lactose); any condition that makes it difficult for you to digest sucrose (table sugar) or lactose (found in milk and milk products), or liver or kidney disease.
- Tell your doctor if you are pregnant, plan to become pregnant, or are breastfeeding. You should not become pregnant while you are taking voriconazole. You should use effective birth control to prevent pregnancy during your treatment with voriconazole. Talk to your doctor about birth control methods that will work for you. If you become pregnant while taking voriconazole, call your doctor immediately. Voriconazole may harm the fetus.
- If you are having surgery, including dental surgery, tell the doctor or dentist that you are taking voriconazole.
- You should know that voriconazole may cause blurred vision or other problems with your eyesight and may make your eyes sensitive to bright light. Do not drive a car at night while taking voriconazole. Do not drive a car during the day or operate machinery if you have any problems with your vision while you are taking this medication.
- Plan to avoid strong, direct sunlight or unnecessary or prolonged exposure to sunlight and to wear protective clothing, sunglasses, and sunscreen. Voriconazole may make your skin sensitive to sunlight. In some patients who have had a reaction to the sun while on voriconazole, skin cancer has developed. Your doctor may refer to you to a dermatologist (skin doctor) to screen and monitor you for skin cancer during and following treatment with voriconazole.

Dietary Instructions

Unless your doctor tells you otherwise, continue your normal diet.

Missed dose

Take the missed dose as soon as you remember it. However, if it is almost time for the next dose, skip the missed dose and continue your regular dosing schedule. Do not take a double dose to make up for a missed one.

Side Effects

Voriconazole may cause side effects. Tell your doctor if any of these symptoms are severe or do not go away:

- Abnormal vision
- Difficulty seeing colors
- Diarrhea
- Nausea
- Vomiting
- Headache
- Dizziness
- Dry mouth
- Flushing

Terbinafine

Terbinafine is an antifungal medicine. It is used to treat skin infections caused by a fungus (yeast), including:

- Athlete's foot,
- Fungal nail infections,
- Ringworm,
- Jock itch (sometimes called dhobie itch, an infection in the groin area), and
- Pityriasis versicolor (this causes small patches of scaly and discoloured skin, often on your back, chest, upper arms, neck and tummy).

Terbinafine comes as a cream, gel or spray for treating athlete's foot, ringworm, jock itch and pityriasis versicolor. There is also a liquid (solution) for athlete's foot. You can buy these from a pharmacy or supermarket.

It also comes as tablets for treating fungal nail infections and other fungal infections. Your doctor may recommend tablets if they think creams, gels, sprays or solution are not likely to work.

Terbinafine tablets are only available on prescription.

Key Facts

- Many fungal infections get better within 7 days of treatment with terbinafine – nail infections can take 3 months or more.
- When using terbinafine on your skin, the most common side effect is irritation in the area where you apply it.
- If you're taking the tablets, the most common side effects are having a smaller appetite than usual, pain in your joints or muscles, or upset stomach.
- The cream, gel and spray usually start to work within a week, and the tablets can take between 2 weeks and a few months to work.
- Brand names for terbinafine tablets and cream include Lamisil. Brand names for the solution for athlete's foot include Lamisil Once.

Prescription of Terbinafine

Tablets, cream and gel can be prescribed for adults and children aged 1 year and over.

The cream, gel and spray that you can buy in a pharmacy or supermarket is suitable for people aged 16 years or older. The solution is only suitable for adults (18 years or older).

To make sure terbinafine is safe for you, tell your doctor or pharmacist if you:

- Have had an allergic reaction to terbinafine or any other medicines in the past.

To make sure the tablets are safe for you, tell your doctor or pharmacist if you:

- Have ever had liver or kidney problems.
- Are pregnant, trying to get pregnant or are breastfeeding.

Side Effects

Like all medicines, terbinafine can cause side effects, although not everyone gets them.

Side effects usually go away when you stop using or taking the medicine.

Common Side Effects

These common side effects happen in more than 1 in 100 people.

If you're using the cream, gel, spray or solution, talk to your pharmacist or doctor if these side effects bother you or do not go away:

- Peeling or itching skin.

If you're taking the tablets, talk to your doctor or a pharmacist if these side effects bother you or do not go away:

- Rash,

- Headache,
- Diarrhoea,
- Feeling or being sick (nausea or vomiting),
- A smaller appetite than usual,
- Stomach ache,
- Indigestion, and
- Muscle or joint pain.

Serious Side Effects

Some people can have serious side effects when using or taking terbinafine. These happen in less than 1 in 1,000 people.

If you're using the cream, gel, spray or solution, stop using terbinafine and call a doctor straight away if:

- You get an itchy rash with blisters, red raised patches or spots (hives), which starts to spread.

If you're prescribed tablets, stop taking them and call a doctor immediately if:

- You get yellow skin or the whites of your eyes turn yellow or if you have pale poo and dark pee – these can be signs of liver problems.
- You bruise more easily or get infections more easily – these can be signs of a blood disorder.
- You have a high temperature with a rash, itchy skin and unusual tiredness, or if you notice any purple spots under your skin – these can be signs of an inflammation of the blood vessels called vasculitis.
- You get severe pain near the top of your stomach that spreads to your back – this can be a sign of an inflamed pancreas.
- Your muscles feel weak or painful, or your pee is a dark red-brown – these can be signs of muscle problems.

Caspofungin

Caspofungin is an antifungal medicine that fights infections caused by fungus. Caspofungin is used to treat fungal infections of the stomach, lungs, esophagus, or other internal body areas. Caspofungin may also be used for purposes not listed in this medication guide.

Warnings

Follow all directions on your medicine label and package. Tell each of your healthcare providers about all your medical conditions, allergies, and all medicines you use.

Precautions before Taking Caspofungin

You should not use caspofungin if you are allergic to it.

Tell your doctor if you have ever had:

- Liver disease, or
- An allergic reaction.

It is not known whether caspofungin will harm an unborn baby. Tell your doctor if you are pregnant.

It may not be safe to breast-feed while using caspofungin. Ask your doctor about any risk.

Using Caspofungin

Caspofungin is given as an infusion into a vein. A healthcare provider will give your first dose and may teach you how to properly use the medication by yourself.

Read and carefully follow any Instructions for Use provided with your medicine. Do not use caspofungin if you don't understand all instructions for proper use. Ask your doctor or pharmacist if you have questions.

Caspofungin must be mixed with a liquid (diluent) before using it. Use only the liquid diluent you have been given to mix with caspofungin. Do not use liquids that contain dextrose or glucose.

Prepare your injection only when you are ready to give it. Do not use if the medicine looks cloudy, has changed colors, or has particles in it. Call your pharmacist for new medicine.

Caspofungin must be given slowly, and the IV infusion can take at least 1 hour to complete.

Caspofungin is usually given for at least 14 days. You may need to receive this medicine until it has been at least 7 days after your symptoms disappear, or 14 days after lab tests show that the infection has cleared.

Use this medicine for the full prescribed length of time, even if your symptoms quickly improve. Skipping doses can increase your risk of infection that is resistant to medication.

You may be given other medications to help treat your infection. Keep using these medicines for as long as your doctor has prescribed.

Use a needle and syringe only once and then place them in a puncture-proof "sharps" container. Follow state or local laws about how to dispose of this container. Keep it out of the reach of children and pets.

Store caspofungin powder in a refrigerator. Do not freeze. You may take the powder out of the refrigerator and allow it to reach room temperature before mixing your medicine.

Flucytosine

Flucytosine is an antifungal medication that fights infections caused by fungus. Flucytosine is used to treat serious fungal infections of the blood, lungs, heart, central nervous system, and urinary tract. Flucytosine is sometimes given with another medicine called amphotericin B. Flucytosine may also be used for purposes not listed here.

Warnings

Before you take flucytosine, tell your doctor if you have kidney disease.

Precautions before Taking Flucytosine

You should not use flucytosine if you are allergic to it.

To make sure flucytosine is safe for you, tell your doctor if you have:

- Kidney disease,
- A blood cell disorder or bone marrow disease,
- Weak immune system (caused by radiation or by using medicine that causes bone marrow suppression), or
- An electrolyte imbalance (such as low levels of potassium in your blood).

It is not known whether flucytosine will harm an unborn baby. Tell your doctor if you are pregnant or plan to become pregnant.

It is not known whether flucytosine passes into breast milk or if it could harm a nursing baby. You should not breast-feed while using this medicine.

Using Flucytosine

Follow all directions on your prescription label. Do not take this medicine in larger or smaller amounts or for longer than recommended.

While using flucytosine, you may need frequent blood tests.

Take each dose with a full glass (8 ounces) of water.

Flucytosine may cause nausea and vomiting. If you take more than one capsule per dose, swallow one capsule at a time over a 15-minute period to help prevent nausea and vomiting.

Use this medicine for the full prescribed length of time. Your symptoms may improve before the infection is completely cleared. Skipping doses may also increase your risk of further infection that is resistant to antifungal medicine. Flucytosine will not treat a viral infection such as the flu or a common cold.

Store at room temperature away from moisture and heat.

Missed dose

Take the missed dose as soon as you remember. Skip the missed dose if it is almost time for your next scheduled dose. Do not take extra medicine to make up the missed dose.

Overdose

Overdose symptoms may include nausea, vomiting, diarrhea, upper stomach pain, or unusual bleeding or bruising.

Precaution

Follow your doctor's instructions about any restrictions on food, beverages, or activity.

Side Effects of Flucytosine

Get emergency medical help if you have signs of an allergic reaction: hives; difficult breathing; swelling of your face, lips, tongue, or throat.

Flucytosine may cause serious side effects. Call your doctor at once if you have:

- Slow heart rate, weak pulse, fainting, slow breathing,
- Chest pain,
- Confusion, hallucinations,
- A seizure (convulsions),
- Pale skin, easy bruising, unusual bleeding (nose, mouth, vagina, or rectum),
- Sudden weakness or ill feeling, fever, chills, sore throat, mouth sores, red or swollen gums, trouble swallowing,
- Problems with hearing,
- Low potassium--leg cramps, constipation, irregular heartbeats, fluttering in your chest, increased thirst or urination, numbness or tingling, muscle weakness or limp feeling,
- Kidney problems--little or no urination, painful or difficult urination, swelling in your feet or ankles, feeling tired or short of breath, or
- Liver problems--nausea, upper stomach pain, itching, tiredness, loss of appetite, dark urine, clay-colored stools, jaundice (yellowing of the skin or eyes).

Common side effects of flucytosine may include:

- Nausea, vomiting, loss of appetite, diarrhea,
- Headache, dizziness,
- Numbness, tingling, or burning pain in your hands or feet,
- Dry mouth, or
- Skin rash.

This is not a complete list of side effects and others may occur. Call your doctor for medical advice about side effects.

Drug Interactions

Tell your doctor about all your current medicines and any you start or stop using, especially:

- Clozapine,
- Cytosine, or
- Deferiprone.

This list is not complete. Other drugs may interact with flucytosine, including prescription and over-the-counter medicines, vitamins, and herbal products. Not all possible interactions are listed here.

Micafungin

Micafungin is an antifungal medication that fights infections caused by fungus. Micafungin is used to treat infections caused by the *Candida* fungus. Micafungin is also used to prevent *Candida* fungal infections in stem cell transplant patients. Micafungin is for use in adults and children who are at least 4 months old.

Micafungin may also be used for purposes not listed here.

Warnings

Follow all directions on your medicine label and package. Tell each of your healthcare providers about all your medical conditions, allergies, and all medicines you use.

Precautions before Taking Micafungin

You should not use this medication if you are allergic to micafungin or similar medicines such as caspofungin (Cancidas) or anidulafungin (Eraxis).

To make sure you can safely use micafungin, tell your doctor if you have any of these other conditions:

- Liver disease, or
- Kidney disease.

It is not known whether micafungin will harm an unborn baby. Tell your doctor if you are pregnant or plan to become pregnant while using this medication.

It is not known whether micafungin passes into breast milk or if it could harm a nursing baby. Tell your doctor if you are breast-feeding a baby.

Using Micafungin

Micafungin is usually given once daily for up to several weeks. Follow all directions on your prescription label. Do not use micafungin in larger or smaller amounts or for longer than recommended.

Micafungin is injected into a vein through an IV. You may be shown how to use an IV at home. Do not self-inject this medicine if you do not understand how to give the injection and properly dispose of used needles, IV tubing, and other items used to inject the medicine.

Do not shake the medication bottle or you may ruin the medicine. Prepare your dose only when you are ready to give an injection. Do not use if the medicine has changed colors or has particles in it. Call your pharmacist for new medicine.

Micafungin must be mixed with a liquid (diluent) before using it. If you are using the injections at home, be sure you understand how to properly mix and store the medicine.

After mixing this medicine, do not expose it to light. Cover the IV bag during your infusion to protect the medicine from light. Use the medicine within 24 hours after mixing.

Micafungin must be given slowly through an IV infusion, and each injection can take at least 1 hour to complete. Do not mix micafungin with any other medicines, or give other medicines through the same IV line.

If a child is using this medication, tell your doctor if the child has any changes in weight. Micafungin doses are based on weight in children.

Use each disposable needle only one time. Throw away used needles in a puncture-proof container (ask your pharmacist where you can get one and how to dispose of it). Keep this container out of the reach of children and pets.

Each single-use vial (bottle) of this medicine is for one use only. Throw away after one use, even if there is still some medicine left in it after injecting your dose.

Store at room temperature away from moisture, heat and light. Mixed medicine can be stored at room temperature but must be used within 24 hours after mixing.

Nystatin

Nystatin is an antifungal medicine. It's used to treat or prevent infections caused by a fungus (or yeast). These include:

- Oral thrush, and
- Skin infections.

Nystatin kills the fungus and gets rid of the infection. It can also be used to stop you getting an infection.

Nystatin is only available on prescription. It comes as a liquid (suspension) that you swirl around your mouth and then swallow. It also comes mixed with steroids, antiseptics or antibacterials as a cream or ointment.

Key Facts

- You usually take nystatin liquid 4 times a day after meals and before bedtime.

- It's important not to eat or drink for 30 minutes after taking the liquid.
- Nystatin usually starts to work after 2 days.
- It's important to continue to take or use nystatin for 2 days after your condition is better. This will help to stop it coming back again.
- Creams and ointments containing nystatin are known by the brand names Trimovate, Timodine or Nystaform HC.

Warnings

Most adults and children, including babies, can take nystatin liquid or use nystatin cream and ointments.

Nystatin is not suitable for everyone. To make sure nystatin is safe for you, tell a pharmacist or doctor if:

- You have ever had an allergic reaction to nystatin or any other medicine in the past (including any ingredients in the cream or ointment).
- You cannot digest some sugars – the liquid has a small amount of sucrose in it.
- You have tuberculosis (TB) of the skin – you may not be able to use the cream or ointment.

Using Nystatin

It's important to take the medicine for as long as your doctor recommends. If you stop taking it too soon, the infection can come back.

Dosage for Nystatin Liquid

The usual dose (for adults, babies and children) to:

- Treat oral thrush is 1ml, taken 4 times a day. Leave at least 3 hours between doses. If your doctor recommends something different, follow their advice.
- Prevent oral thrush is 1ml, taken once or twice a day.

Using Nystatin Liquid

People usually take nystatin liquid for around 1 week to treat oral thrush.

It's best to take it after a meal or some food. However, do not mix it with food or water or any other drink.

1. Shake the bottle well.
2. Take the lid off and measure out the right amount using an oral syringe, medicine spoon or dropper. Do not use a kitchen teaspoon as it will not give you the right amount.
3. Put the medicine in your mouth.

4. Keep it in your mouth for at least 30 seconds if possible, using it like a mouthwash before you swallow it.
5. Do not eat or drink anything for 30 minutes after taking it. This stops you washing the medicine out of your mouth too soon.

It may be difficult to get your child to keep it in their mouth, but encourage them to do this if you can. Do not worry if they cannot. The medicine will still help even if they swallow it quickly.

Nystatin Cream or Ointment

Nystatin is also available in creams and ointments mixed with other ingredients. Your doctor will decide which is best for you.

You will usually apply a cream or ointment 2 or 3 times a day, for a maximum of 7 days. The amount you use will depend on the skin condition you have. Your doctor or pharmacist will tell you how much to use and how long to use it for.

Missed dose

If you forget a dose, take it as soon as you remember, unless it's nearly time for your next dose. In this case, just skip the missed dose and take your next one as normal.

Do not take a double dose to make up for a missed dose.

If you forget doses often, it may help to set an alarm to remind you. You could also ask your pharmacist for advice on other ways to remember your medicines.

Excessive dose

Nystatin is generally very safe. Taking too much is unlikely to harm you or your child.

If you're worried, speak to your pharmacist or doctor.

If your nystatin cream or ointment contains a strong steroid called clobetasol, talk to your pharmacist or doctor. They'll be able to tell you if you've used too much.

Side Effects of Nystatin

Like all medicines, nystatin can cause side effects, but most people have no side effects or only minor ones.

Common Side Effects

If you're taking nystatin liquid, talk to your pharmacist or doctor if these side effects bother you or do not go away:

- Diarrhoea, and
- Feeling or being sick (nausea or vomiting).

If you're using nystatin cream or ointment, stop using the product and talk to your pharmacist or doctor if:

- You have a rash or itchy, dry or swollen skin where you have applied it.
- You get a new infection.

Your pharmacist or doctor may be able to recommend a different medicine.

Serious Allergic Reaction

It happens rarely but it is possible to have a serious allergic reaction (anaphylaxis) to nystatin.

Natamycin

NATAMYCIN belongs to a class of medication called 'antifungal' used to treat fungal infections of the eye. A fungal infection is a disease in which a fungus attacks the tissue and causes damage to the eye. Fungi are commonly present in nature but do not cause infections normally. However, if the fungi enter the eye, then it causes eye pain, redness, and blurred vision.

NATAMYCIN contains 'Natamycin', which works by killing fungi by destroying their outer cell membrane. The fungal cell membranes are essential for their survival as they prevent the entry of unwanted substances into the cells and stop the leakage of cell contents.

Use NATAMYCIN as suggested by the doctor. You are advised to use NATAMYCIN for as long as your doctor has prescribed it for you based on your medical condition. In some cases, you may experience eye irritation, allergic reaction, vision change and eye pain. Most of these side effects of NATAMYCIN do not require medical attention and gradually resolve over time. However, if the side effects persist or worsen, please consult your doctor.

Before using NATAMYCIN, tell your doctor if you have any allergy to any of its components. NATAMYCIN should only be used in pregnancy or breastfeeding females if specified by the doctor. NATAMYCIN is not recommended for children as safety and effectiveness were not established. Avoid driving after taking NATAMYCIN as it may affect your ability to drive. NATAMYCIN is safe to use in elderly people as no difference in safety and effectiveness has been observed.

Use of NATAMYCIN:

- Fungal eye infection

Medicinal Benefits

NATAMYCIN is recommended for the treatment of fungal infections of the eye such as conjunctivitis (infection of the white part of the eye), endophthalmitis (infection of the inside part of the eye) and keratitis (infection of the clear part of the eye) caused by fungi in the eyes. It acts by stopping the growth of fungus in the eye that provides relief in irritation, redness, itching, swelling of the eye associated with a fungal eye infection.

Directions for Use

NATAMYCIN is only for external use. Lie down and tilt your head backward. Pull your lower eyelid gently with your index finger to form a pocket. Instil the number of drops advised by the doctor into the pocket of the lower eyelid. Close your eyes for 1-2 minutes. Do not touch the tip of the dropper as it may contaminate the contents. Do not place the tip directly into the eye while instilling drops. If the dropper touches the eye, immediately squeeze two to three drops onto the tissue and wipe the dropper's tip with salt water.

Storage

Store in a cool and dry place away from sunlight

Side Effects of NATAMYCIN

- Mild eye discomfort,
- Change in vision,
- Allergic reaction,
- Chest pain,
- Eye swelling, and
- Eye pain.

Echinocandins

Echinocandins are a new class of antifungals and are water-soluble cyclic lipopeptides (lipid connected to a peptide) that inhibit glucan synthase. They are used to treat invasive fungal infections and show good activity against amphotericin B-resistant and fluconazole-resistant *Candida guilliermondii.*

Echinocandins work by inhibiting a glucosyltransferase enzyme (1→3)-β-D-glucan synthase, which is essential for the generation of (1→3)-β-D-glucan, an essential component that maintains the integrity of the fungal cell wall. The inability of the organism to synthesize (1→3)-β-D-glucan leads to osmotic instability and cell death. The spectrum of activity of echinocandins is limited to pathogens that rely on these glucan polymers and is less broad than the spectrums of other antifungals such as the polyene or azole agents. Mammalian cells have no cell wall, so echinocandins have very few toxic adverse effects in humans.

Echinocandins exhibit fungistatic activity (inhibit the growth of fungus) against aspergillosis species, whereas they exhibit fungicidal activity (kill parasitic fungi or their spores) against *Candida* species.

Using Echinocandin Antifungals

Echinocandin antifungals are administered only by the intravenous route to treat:

- Esophageal candidiasis (the most common type of infectious esophagitis).

- Invasive candidiasis (an infection caused by a yeast [a type of fungus] called Candida).
- Candidemia (a Candida bloodstream infection).
- Invasive aspergillosis (an infection of the pulmonary, parenchyma, which is affected by the growing hyphae of Aspergillus).
- Empirical therapy in febrile neutropenia.

Side Effects of Echinocandin Antifungals

Side effects of echinocandin antifungals may include:

- Facial flushing (temporary reddening of the skin because of dilation of blood vessels beneath the skin),
- Severe rash,
- Itching,
- Fever,
- Thrombophlebitis (inflammation of a vein, usually in the leg), and
- Hepatitis (inflammation of the liver).

Mechanism and Site of Action of Antifungal Drugs

The two main mechanisms of action of antifungals targeting the cell wall are related to the inhibition of chitin and β-glucan synthesis.

An understanding of the mechanisms of action and in vitro profiles of antifungal agents is pivotal to selecting effective treatments for dermatophytoses. The principal mechanisms of action of antifungal drugs include disruption of spindle and cytoplasmic microtubule function (e.g., griseofulvin), depletion of or binding to ergosterol (e.g., terbinafine, ketoconazole, and amphotericin B), and accumulation of squalene (terbinafine). It is likely that antifungal agents that deplete or bind to ergosterol have fungistatic activity only; agents that produce a concomitant accumulation of intracellular squalene have fungicidal activity. Although the mechanism of action markedly influences the clinical efficacy of an antifungal agent, in vitro and in vivo antimycotic profiles and bioavailability factors such as drug access to the stratum corneum also contribute to the effectiveness of antifungal agents.

Emerging Novel Antifungals

Keeping in view the facts that there are limited antifungal strategies and paucity of effective drugs, there is continuous hunt for the development of novel and effective antifungals to combat the fungal infections. Many different drug categories which show promising antifungal activity are at various stages of the development.

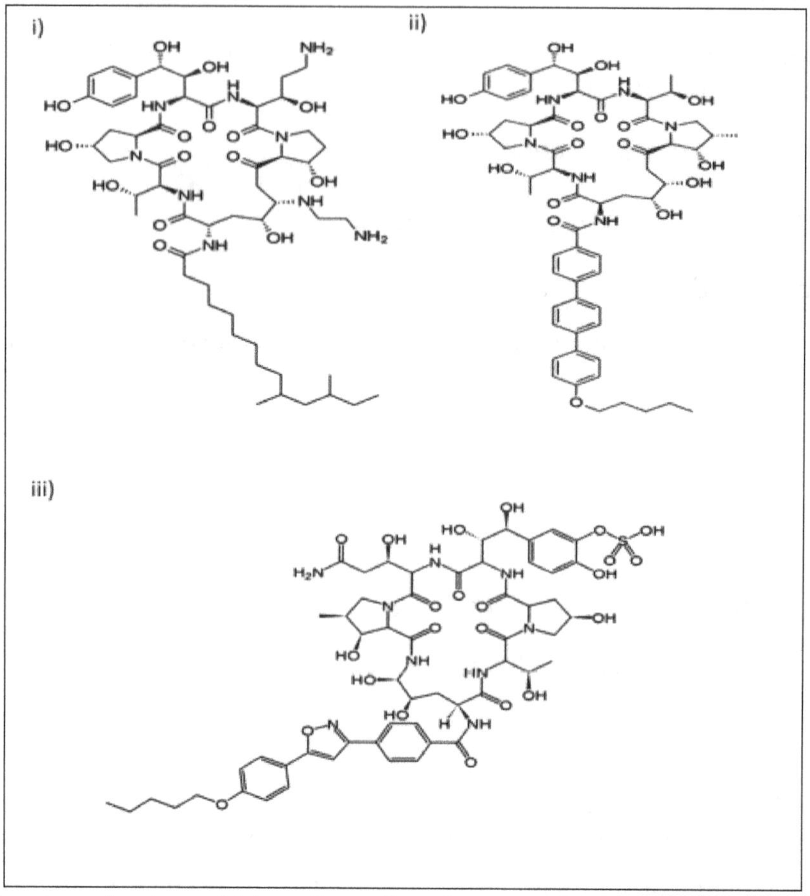

Figure: Structure of various echinocandin antifungal compounds targeting unique components in fungal CW. These include (i) Caspofungin (ii) Anidulafungin and (iii) Micafungin

Resistance against Antifungal Drugs

Antifungal resistance occurs when an antifungal medication no longer works to treat a fungal infection. The fungus can fight off the medicine's effects.

This problem is a type of antimicrobial resistance. It occurs when fungi, viruses, bacteria and parasites don't respond to medications developed to treat them. Your body doesn't develop antifungal resistance — fungi do. Today, while antifungal medicines may still help you, fewer drugs can treat drug-resistant fungi.

Antifungal Medications

Antifungal drugs help your body get rid of certain fungal infections. They treat fungal skin infections like yeast infections, athlete's foot, jock itch and ringworm. Antifungal medicines also manage infections that affect the lungs, brain and blood.

Problem of Antifungal Resistance

Drug resistance is a serious global health problem. It greatly limits treatment options. If a fungus doesn't respond to one of three available classes of antifungal drugs, the other options may be less effective. Some drugs cause more severe, potentially toxic side effects.

Nearly 3 million Americans will develop a drug-resistant infection this year. More than 35,000 of them will die.

Causes of Antifungal Resistance

There are several causes of antifungal resistance:

- Improper use of antifungal medicines: When you skip doses, stop treatment too soon or receive a dose that's too low, a fungus gets better at fighting off the medicine's effects.
- Antibiotic use: Antibiotics kill harmful bacteria. But they can also kill helpful bacteria in the digestive tract. As a result, Candida, a yeast naturally found inside the digestive tract, can start to grow too fast. A person taking antibiotics may then need antifungals to treat a yeast infection called candidiasis. Frequent treatment raises the risk of drug resistance to both treatments.
- Fungicide use: People who work closely with crops treated by fungicides may be more prone to fungal infections that are antifungal-resistant. In these environments, fungi have increased exposure to fungicides. Fungicides are a type of antifungal that keeps crops from getting moldy.
- Natural resistance: Certain fungi never respond to antifungals. They're naturally resistant to medicines.
- Spontaneous resistance: A fungus stops responding to a once-effective medicine for no known reason.
- Transmitted resistance: You can spread a contagious drug-resistant fungal infection to someone else. That person now has an infection that won't respond to an antifungal, even if they've never used the medicine.

People Susceptible to Antifungal Resistance

People who have weakened immune systems are more likely to develop serious fungal infections that can lead to antifungal resistance. This includes people who have:

- AIDS,
- Autoimmune diseases like lupus,
- Cancer,
- Organ transplants, and
- Stem cell (bone marrow) transplants.

Complications of Antifungal Resistance

Certain strains of fungi have become more resistant to antifungal medicines. They're known as superbugs. These fungi continue to multiply and cause infections even when you take medication.

There are only three classes of antifungal medicines: azoles, echinocandin and polyenes. A fungus that develops resistance to one drug may not respond to any available treatments.

Antifungal Superbugs

Fungal infections with superbug status include:

- Aspergillus fumigatus: This mold causes a lung infection called aspergillosis. Approximately 200,000 people worldwide develop aspergillosis every year. They typically get it from breathing in the mold spores. The infection is becoming more resistant to azole antifungals.
- Candida: This yeast naturally occurs on the skin and inside the body. Candida can enter the bloodstream, causing a potentially life-threatening infection called candidemia. This infection no longer responds well to azole medicines.
- Candida glabrata: C. glabrata affects the urinary system. It's becoming more resistant to azoles and echinocandins. That leaves people with few safe treatment options.

Permissions

All chapters in this book are published with permission under the Creative Commons Attribution Share Alike License or equivalent. Every chapter published in this book has been scrutinized by our experts. Their significance has been extensively debated. The topics covered herein carry significant information for a comprehensive understanding. They may even be implemented as practical applications or may be referred to as a beginning point for further studies.

We would like to thank the editorial team for lending their expertise to make the book truly unique. They have played a crucial role in the development of this book. Without their invaluable contributions this book wouldn't have been possible. They have made vital efforts to compile up to date information on the varied aspects of this subject to make this book a valuable addition to the collection of many professionals and students.

This book was conceptualized with the vision of imparting up-to-date and integrated information in this field. To ensure the same, a matchless editorial board was set up. Every individual on the board went through rigorous rounds of assessment to prove their worth. After which they invested a large part of their time researching and compiling the most relevant data for our readers.

The editorial board has been involved in producing this book since its inception. They have spent rigorous hours researching and exploring the diverse topics which have resulted in the successful publishing of this book. They have passed on their knowledge of decades through this book. To expedite this challenging task, the publisher supported the team at every step. A small team of assistant editors was also appointed to further simplify the editing procedure and attain best results for the readers.

Apart from the editorial board, the designing team has also invested a significant amount of their time in understanding the subject and creating the most relevant covers. They scrutinized every image to scout for the most suitable representation of the subject and create an appropriate cover for the book.

The publishing team has been an ardent support to the editorial, designing and production team. Their endless efforts to recruit the best for this project, has resulted in the accomplishment of this book. They are a veteran in the field of academics and their pool of knowledge is as vast as their experience in printing. Their expertise and guidance has proved useful at every step. Their uncompromising quality standards have made this book an exceptional effort. Their encouragement from time to time has been an inspiration for everyone.

The publisher and the editorial board hope that this book will prove to be a valuable piece of knowledge for students, practitioners and scholars across the globe.

Index